PIERRE DELAERE

Replacement and Transplantation of the Larynx and Trachea

LANNOO
CAMPUS

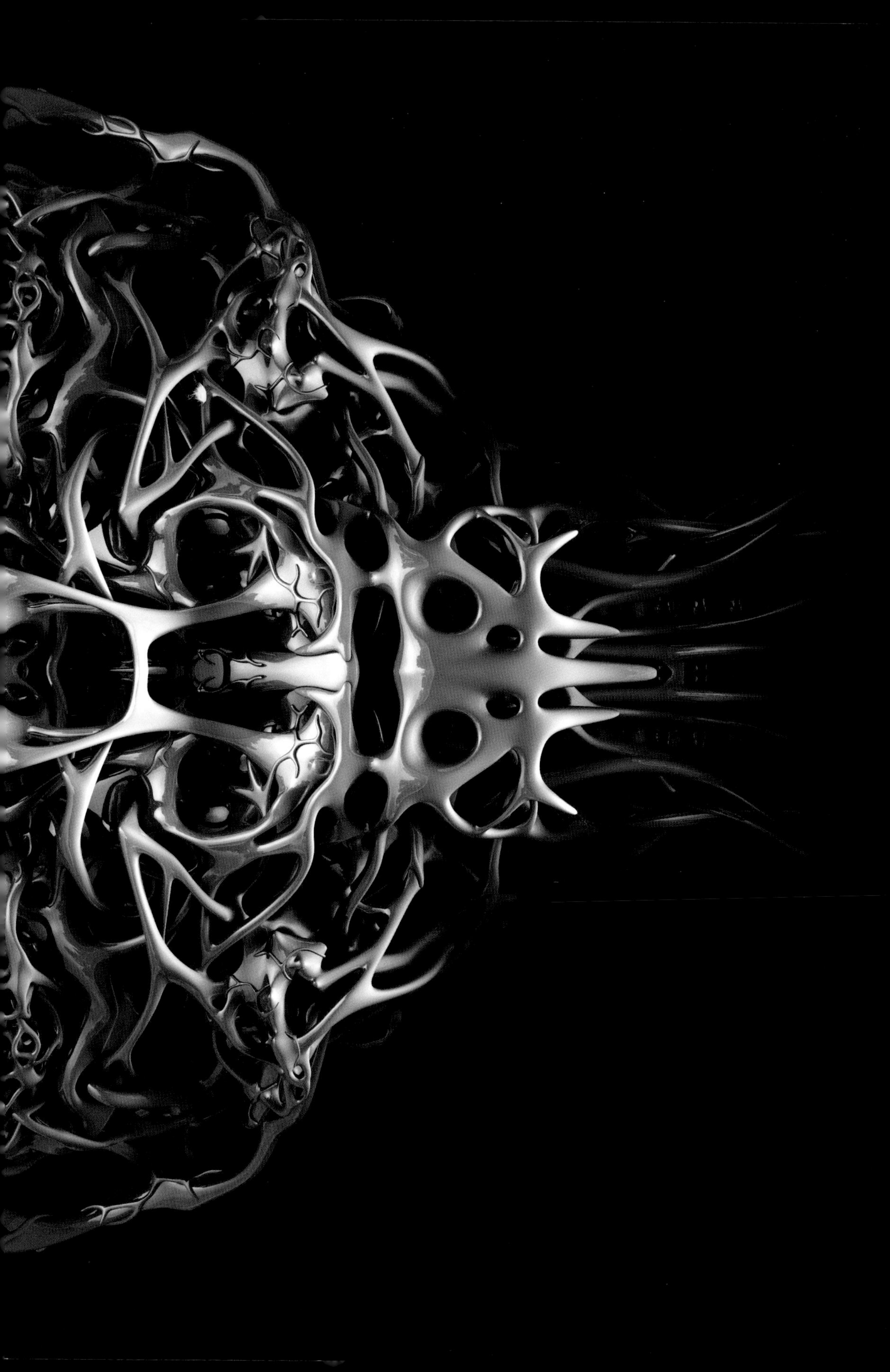

Contents

A personal viewpoint
Where research meets clinical application
Where science meets art

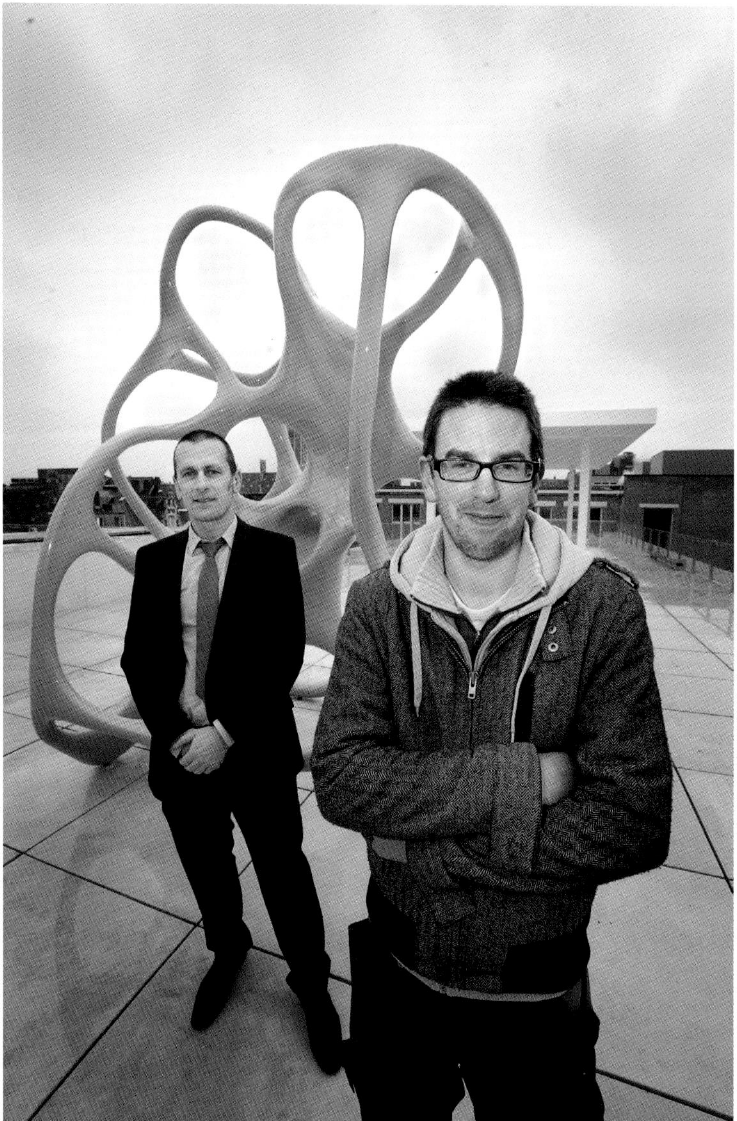

Pierre Delaere Nick Ervinck

(sculpture in background: Niebloy, 2009)

Replacement and Transplantation of the Larynx and Trachea is a visual representation of the current possibilities in laryngotracheal reconstruction. This atlas is principally based on knowledge that has been gathered over a 25-year period of experimental and clinical research at the University of Leuven, Belgium.

In 1988, experimental animal research was started in an attempt to develop improved reconstruction techniques for the larynx and trachea. Using the rabbit as an experimental animal, we sought a well-vascularized tissue that could recreate the cartilaginous support and mucosal lining with preserved viability inside laryngeal and tracheal defects. This experimental model enabled the study of basic airway wound healing mechanisms. The clinical concepts of a mucosal-lined fascial flap, tracheal autotransplantation, and the first clinical cases of vascularized tracheal allotransplantation resulted from these studies.

The emphasis of this atlas lies on the artwork. The medical artwork produced for this publication caught the fascination of Belgium-based artist, Nick Ervinck. In his work, Ervinck often responds to technological challenges in the field of contemporary art, making use of new media and techniques. He creates sculptures that are on the edges of the physical and virtual realms, constantly exploring the limits of the possible. 3D printing, for instance, allows the artist to produce complex forms and shapes that are impossible to sculpt by hand. Ervinck's work has been shown internationally.

Following on from a previous collaboration for 'Parallellipipeda', an exhibition on art and science at the M-Museum, Leuven, Nick Ervinck has created several more pieces inspired by visual imagery from my own medical research. The result of the interaction between the medical field of laryngotracheal repair and Ervinck's artistic universe is visible at the beginning of each chapter.

I must express special thanks to my colleagues who assisted me with the experimental or clinical part of this work. I am thankful to Patrick Meeze who created the beautiful medical artwork throughout the book.

Pierre Delaere

The authors of this book have no conflicts of interest to disclose.

www.kuleuven.be/cltr
www.nickervinck.com

In AGRIEBORZ*, imagery of the upper aerodigestive tract is used as a building material to construct an organic form, a larynx 'gone wild'. As a sculpture, it is impossible to capture in a single glance. There is a visual connection to the upper aerodigestive tract, tracheostoma and capillary networks, etc. Yet a coherent organization is lacking, leaving the viewer with an alienating effect.*

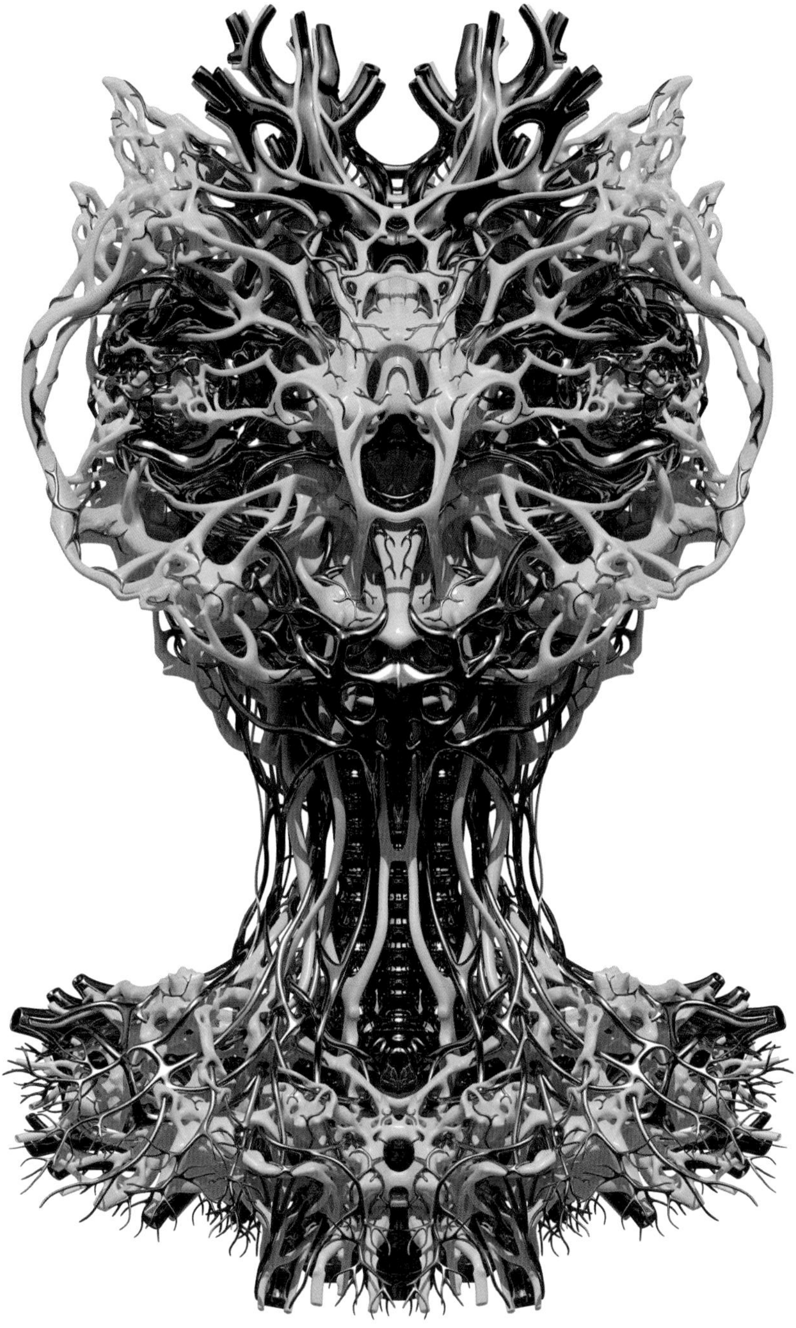

AGRIEBORZ, 2009-2011

LIGHTBOX

200 × 12 × 17 CM

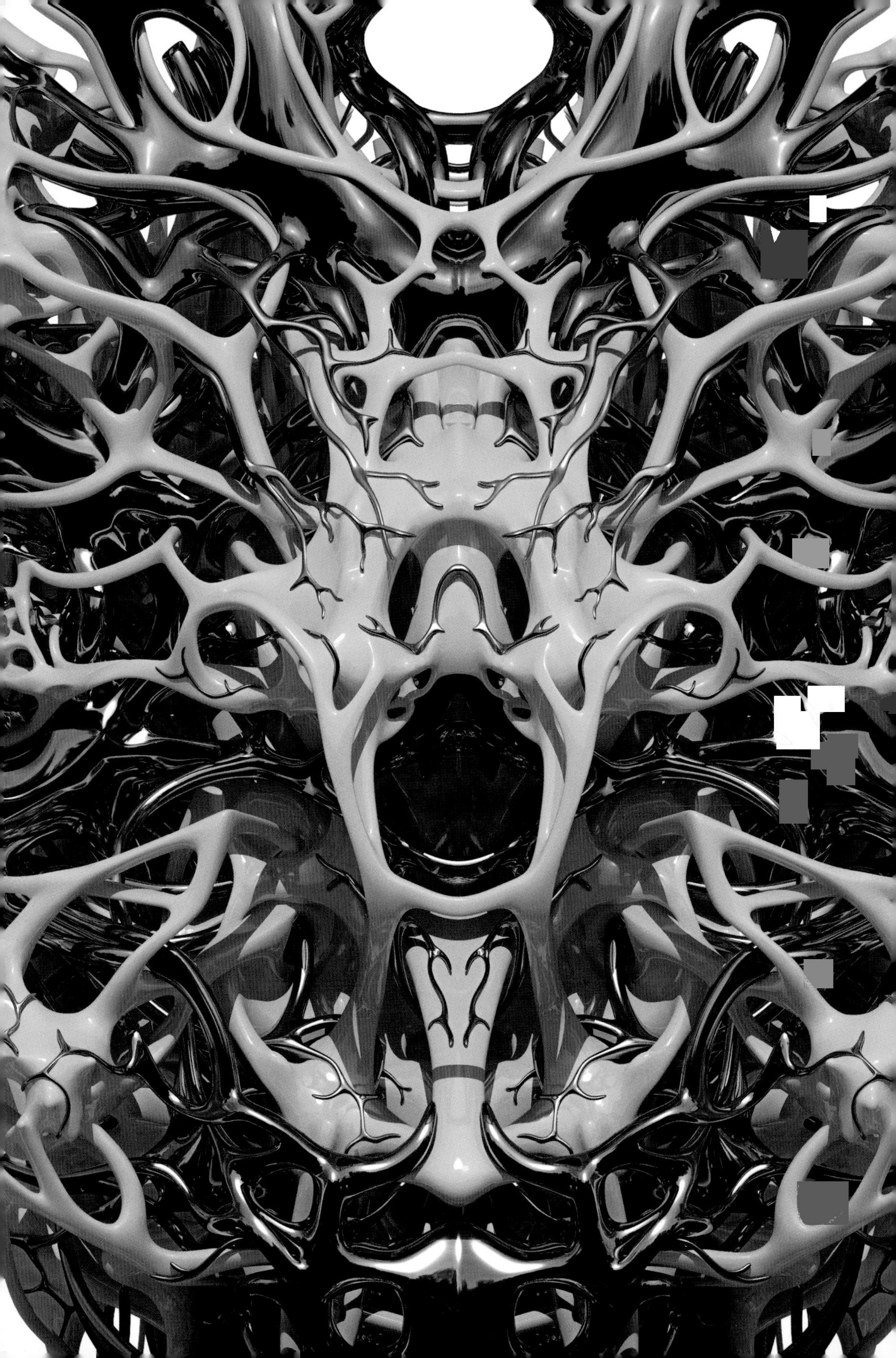

1. Avoiding the use of repair tissue

Secondary healing

Tracheal resection

Cricotracheal resection

Prosthetic replacement: airway versus vascular conduits

Laryngeal or tracheal defects may result after tumor resection or after the excision of stenotic segments. The majority of these defects can be treated without the use of repair tissue. Secondary healing may be the best option after a partial laryngectomy. Bridging of the defect by the anastomosis of the upper and lower resection margins is preferable after tracheal or cricotracheal resection. Prosthetic replacement could also be considered as a possible solution to avoid repair tissues. However, prosthetic airway repair is not possible.

Secondary healing

SURGICAL DEFECTS OF THE SUPRAGLOTTIC AND GLOTTIC AREAS DO NOT REQUIRE THE USE OF REPAIR TISSUE AS MOST CAN HEAL BY SECONDARY INTENTION.

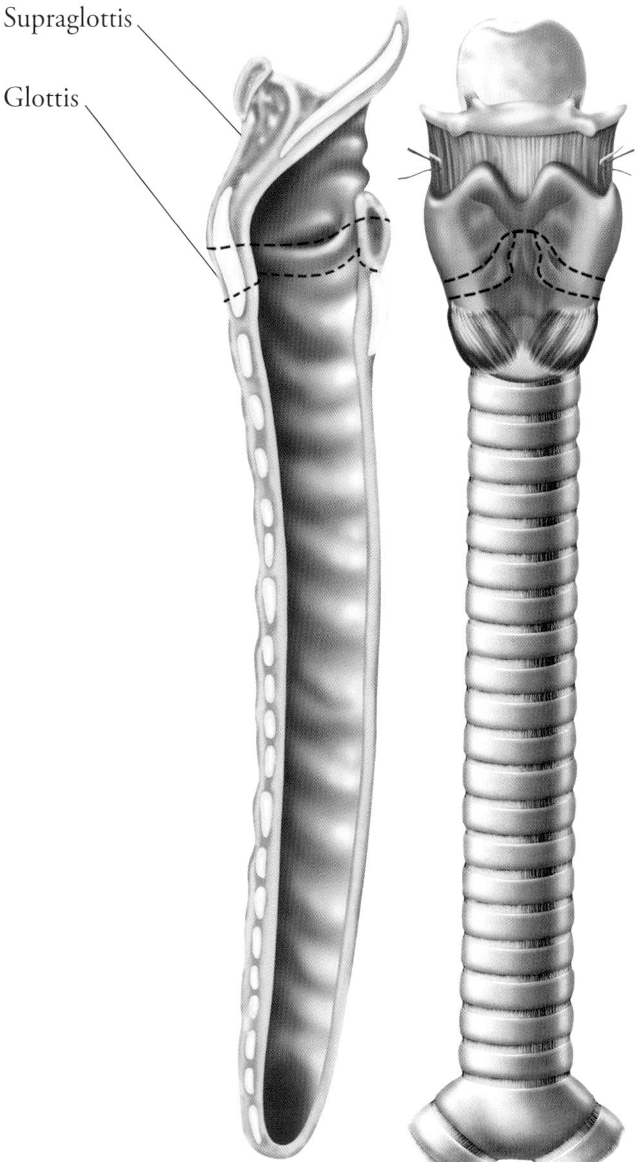
Supraglottis
Glottis

"Most glottic and supraglottic defects can heal by secondary intention without the adverse effects (stenosis) that are typically linked with secondary healing in other parts of the respiratory tract."

Current treatment options for the management of early glottic and supraglotttic carcinoma are endoscopic laser excision or primary radiotherapy. The defects that result after laser excision of a glottic (chordectomy) or supraglottic (supraglottic laryngectomy) tumor heal by secondary intention.

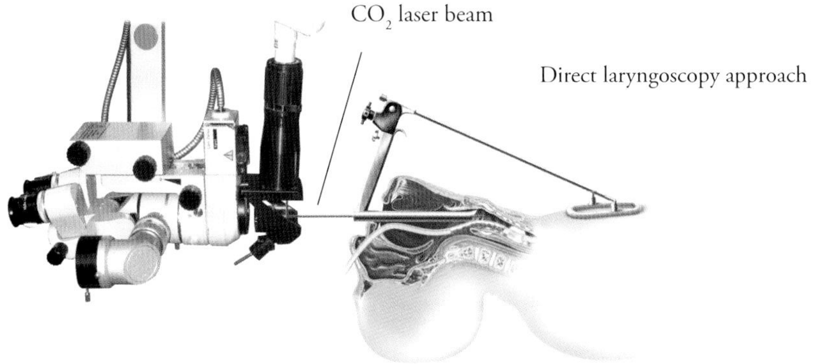
CO_2 laser beam
Direct laryngoscopy approach

CHORDECTOMY

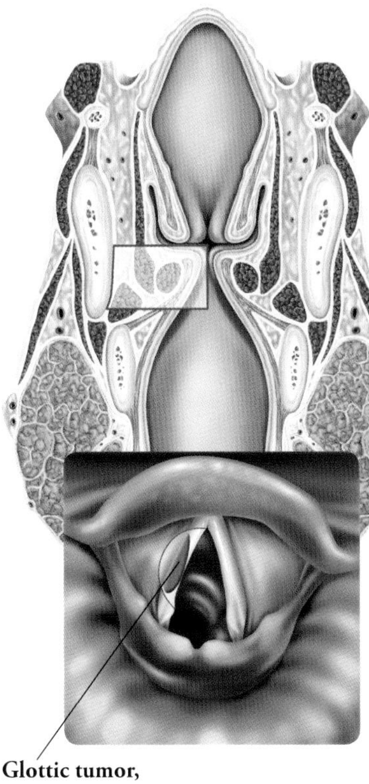

Glottic tumor,
showing the amount of resection.

SUPRAGLOTTIC
LARYNGECTOMY

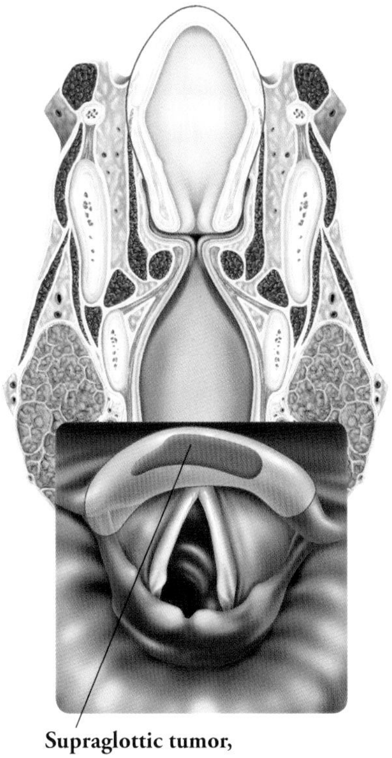

Supraglottic tumor,
showing the amount of resection.

Tracheal resection

A SEGMENTAL AIRWAY RESECTION WITH AN END-TO-END ANASTOMOSIS IS PERFORMED DURING TRACHEAL RESECTION. A TRACHEAL TUMOR OR A TRACHEAL STENOSIS WITH A LENGTH OF LESS THAN 5 CM CAN BE RESECTED WITH AN END-TO-END ANASTOMOSIS.

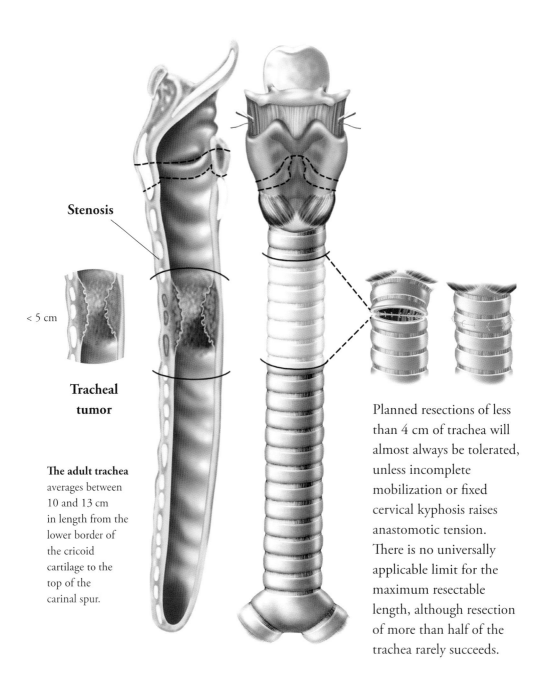

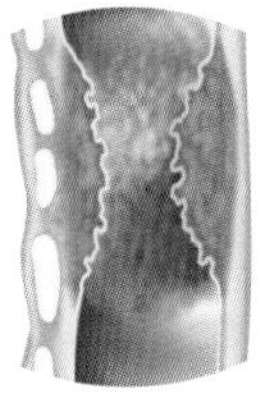
< 5 cm
Tracheal tumor

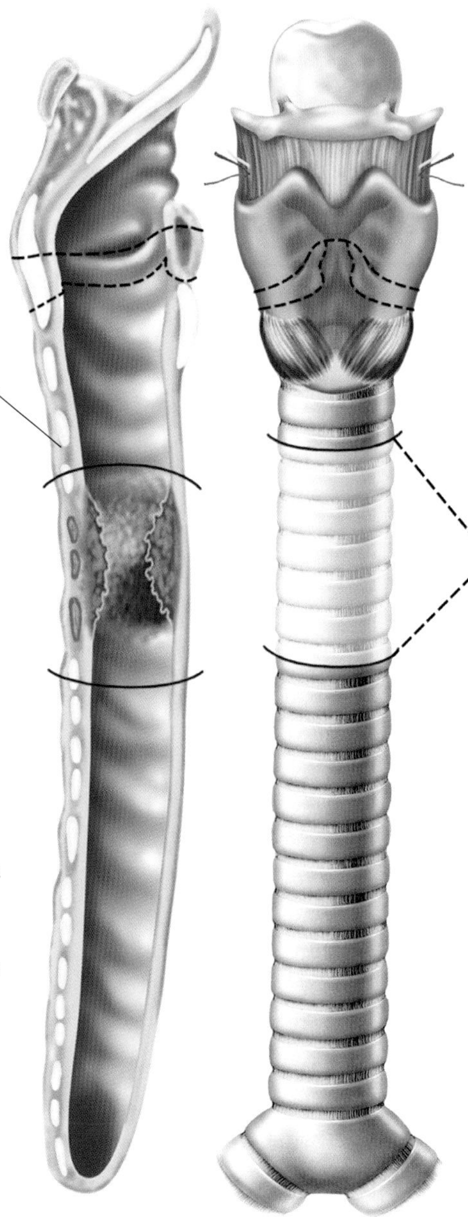
Stenosis

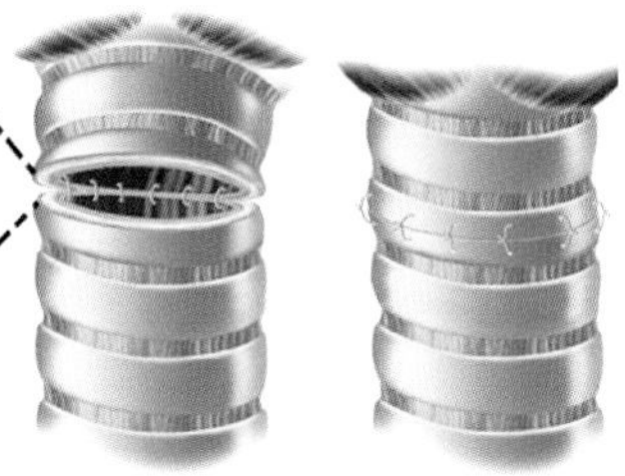

The adult trachea averages between 10 and 13 cm in length from the lower border of the cricoid cartilage to the top of the carinal spur.

Planned resections of less than 4 cm of trachea will almost always be tolerated, unless incomplete mobilization or fixed cervical kyphosis raises anastomotic tension. There is no universally applicable limit for the maximum resectable length, although resection of more than half of the trachea rarely succeeds.

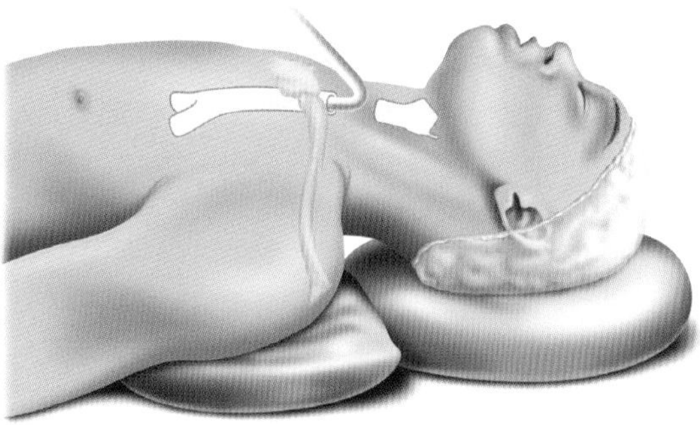

During the resection of the involved segment, the orotracheal tube is replaced with an endotracheal tube through the distal tracheal stump.

During an end-to-end anastomosis, the patient is intubated transorally and the head is brought into flexion.

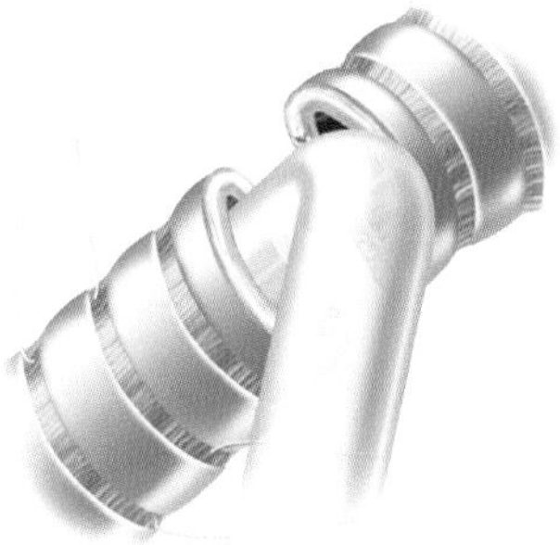

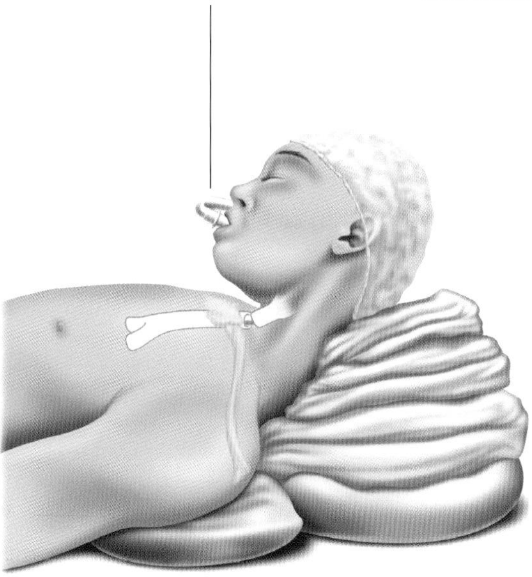

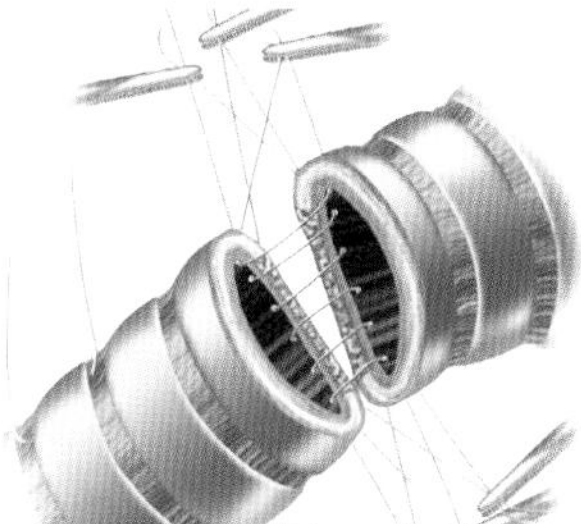

Posterior anastomosis

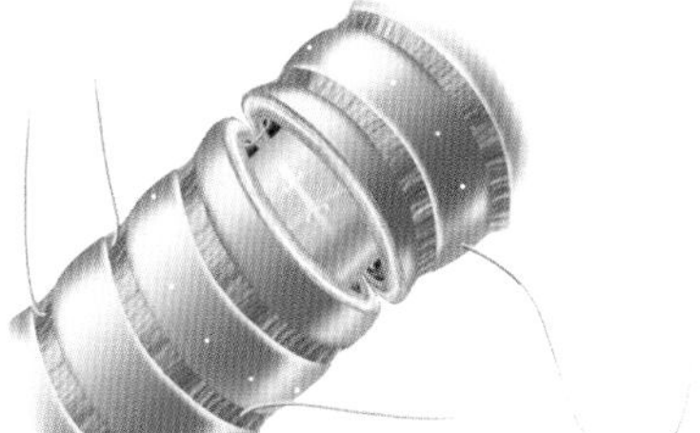

Anterior anastomosis

Cricotracheal resection

CRICOTRACHEAL RESECTION IS MOSTLY ADVOCATED TO RESOLVE A SUBGLOTTIC STENOSIS. CRICOTRACHEAL RESECTION WITH AN ANASTOMOSIS OF THE TRACHEA TO THE THYROID CARTILAGE IS THE TREATMENT OF CHOICE FOR THE CURE OF (IDIOPATHIC) SUBGLOTTIC STENOSIS WITH NORMAL VOCAL FOLD MOBILITY.

Idiopathic subglottic stenosis, showing the amount of resection (cervicotomy approach)

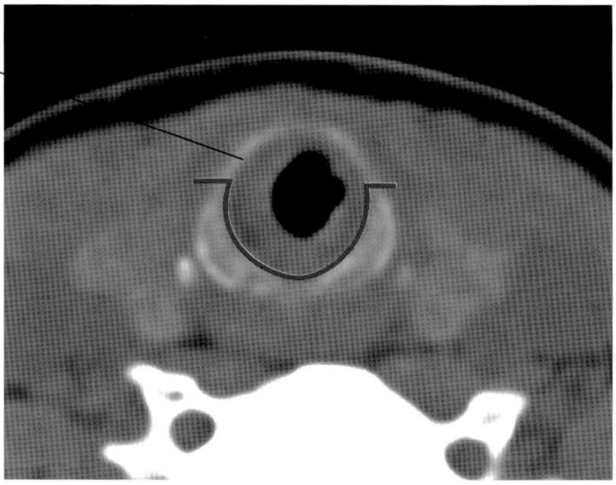

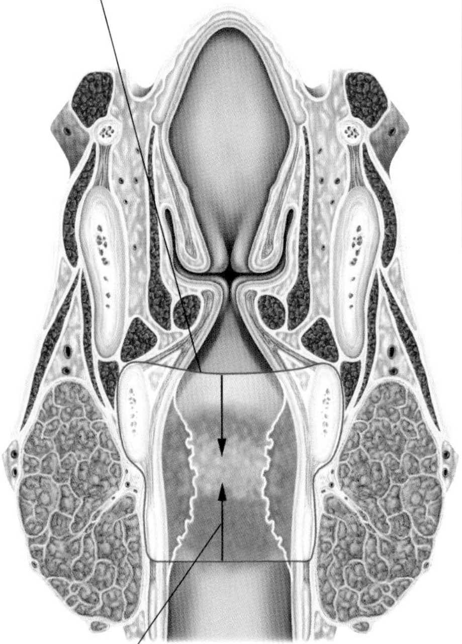

Arrows indicate the anastomosis of the trachea to the thyroid cartilage.

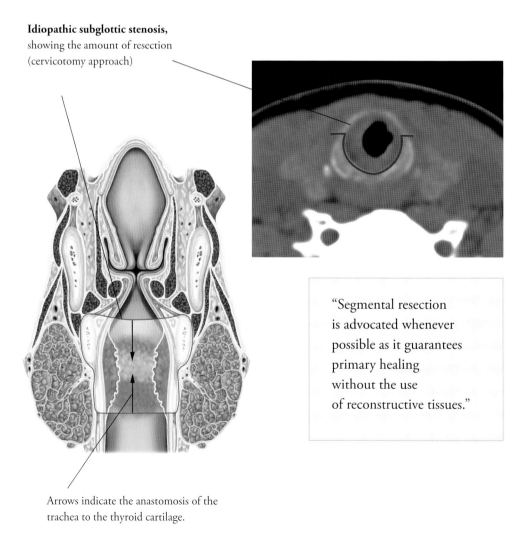

"Segmental resection is advocated whenever possible as it guarantees primary healing without the use of reconstructive tissues."

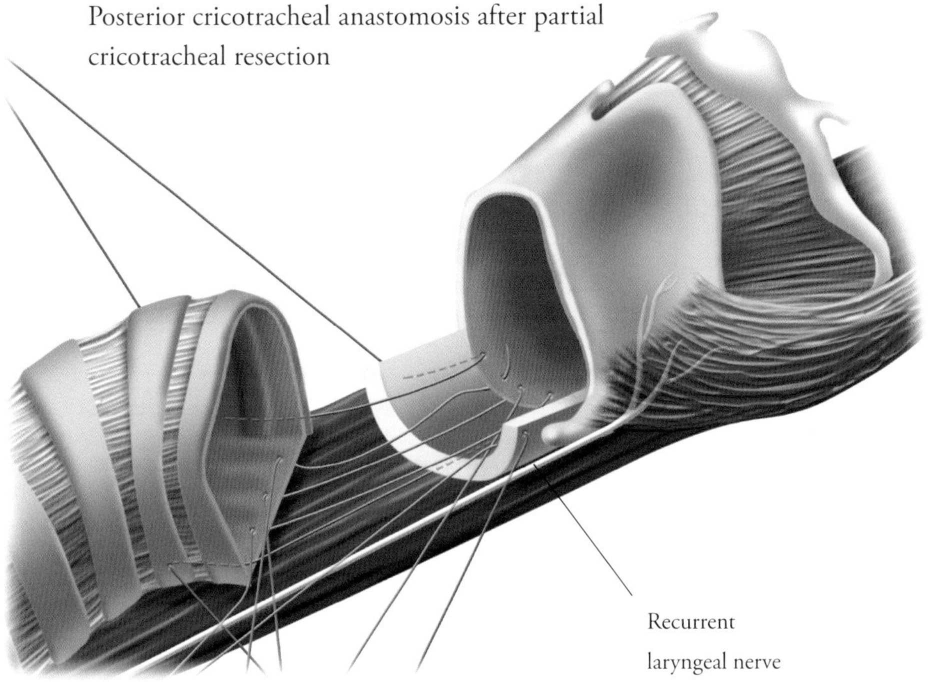
Posterior cricotracheal anastomosis after partial cricotracheal resection
Recurrent laryngeal nerve

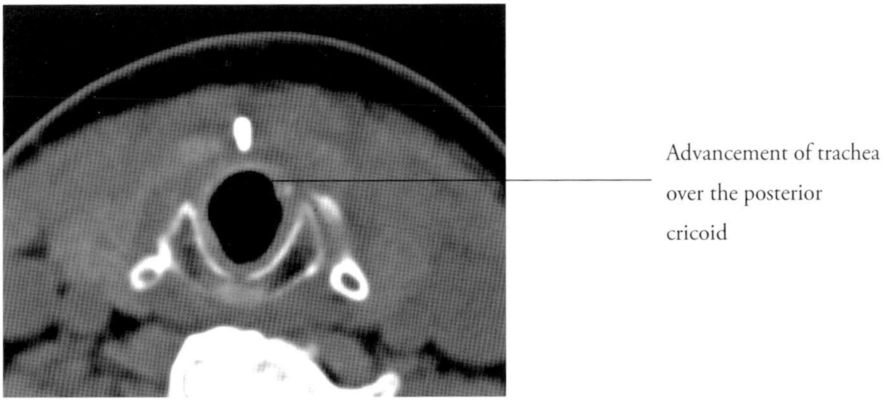
Advancement of trachea over the posterior cricoid

For details, see: Monnier P. Pediatric airway surgery. Springer-Verlag Berlin Heidelberg 2011.

Prosthetic replacement: airway versus vascular conduits

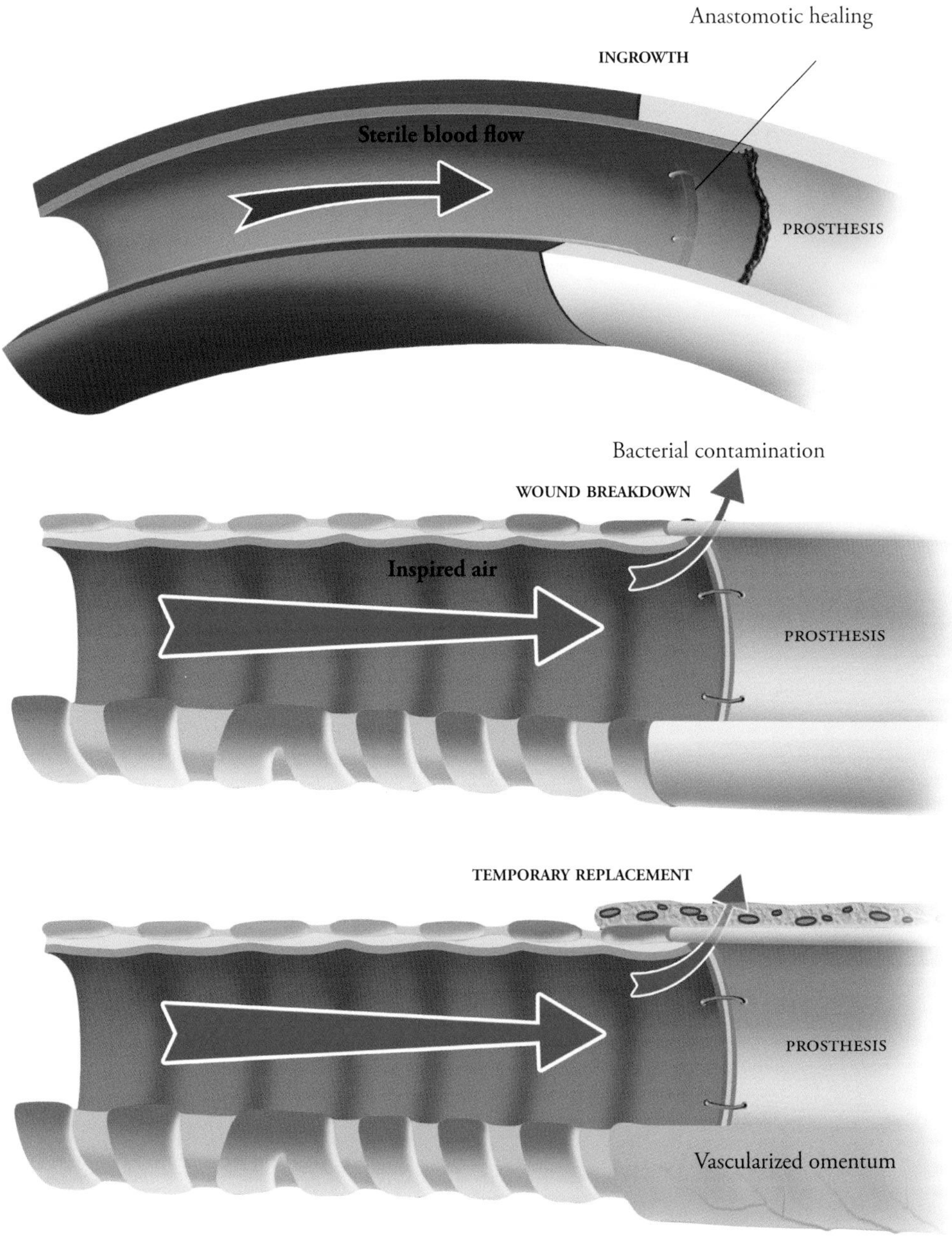
Anastomotic healing
INGROWTH
Sterile blood flow
PROSTHESIS
Bacterial contamination
WOUND BREAKDOWN
Inspired air
PROSTHESIS
TEMPORARY REPLACEMENT
PROSTHESIS
Vascularized omentum

PROSTHETIC REPLACEMENT OF THE AIRWAY IS NOT POSSIBLE. TO DATE, ALL SURGICAL PROSTHESES THAT HAVE BEEN SUCCESSFUL (E.G., VASCULAR CONDUITS) HAVE BEEN SITED IN POTENTIALLY STERILE MESENCHYMAL TISSUES.

BLOOD VESSEL PROSTHESIS

Endothelialization of the luminal surface of vascular grafts occurs only 1 to 2 cm into the graft from the anastomotic site. These endothelial cells are derived from adjacent, native arterial endothelium and they enable the anastomosis to heal.

AIRWAY PROSTHESIS

In the respiratory tract, the flow of inspired air will lead to bacterial contamination and wound breakdown at the anastomoses. The respiratory epithelium will not grow over the prosthesis-airway anastomosis.

"Definitive prosthetic airway repair is not possible."

AIRWAY PROSTHESIS WRAPPED IN VASCULARIZED TISSUE

A prosthesis may act as a temporary airway stent when it is wrapped by well-vascularized tissue (e.g., omentum). The vascularized tissue around the prosthesis may temporarily avoid the complications of wound breakdown at the anastomotic sites. This replacement is comparable to the replacement with a tracheal stent wrapped with a vascularized flap (see page 31).

"As a 'sculptor' I have one foot firmly planted in the digital world. I don't use the computer as a mere instrument, it is rather the digital logic itself that largely determines my artistic thought and method."

NICK ERVINCK

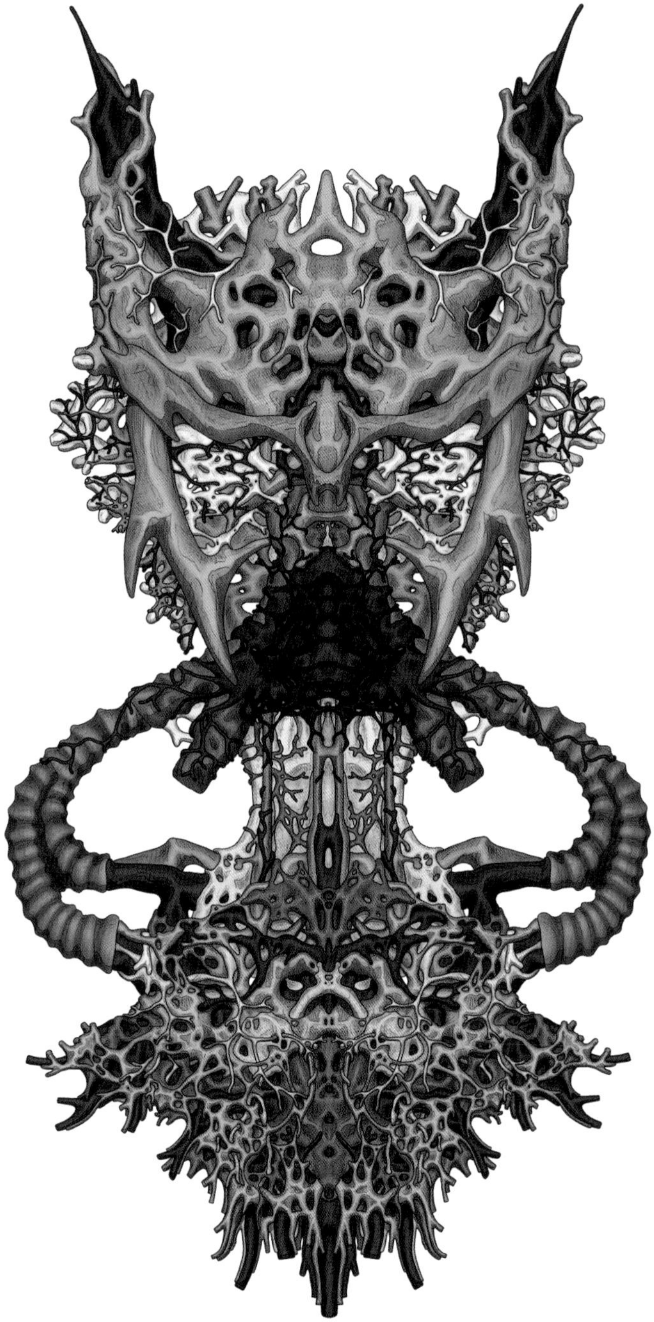

LEKZAORZ, 2010-2011

PRINT

155 × 120 CM

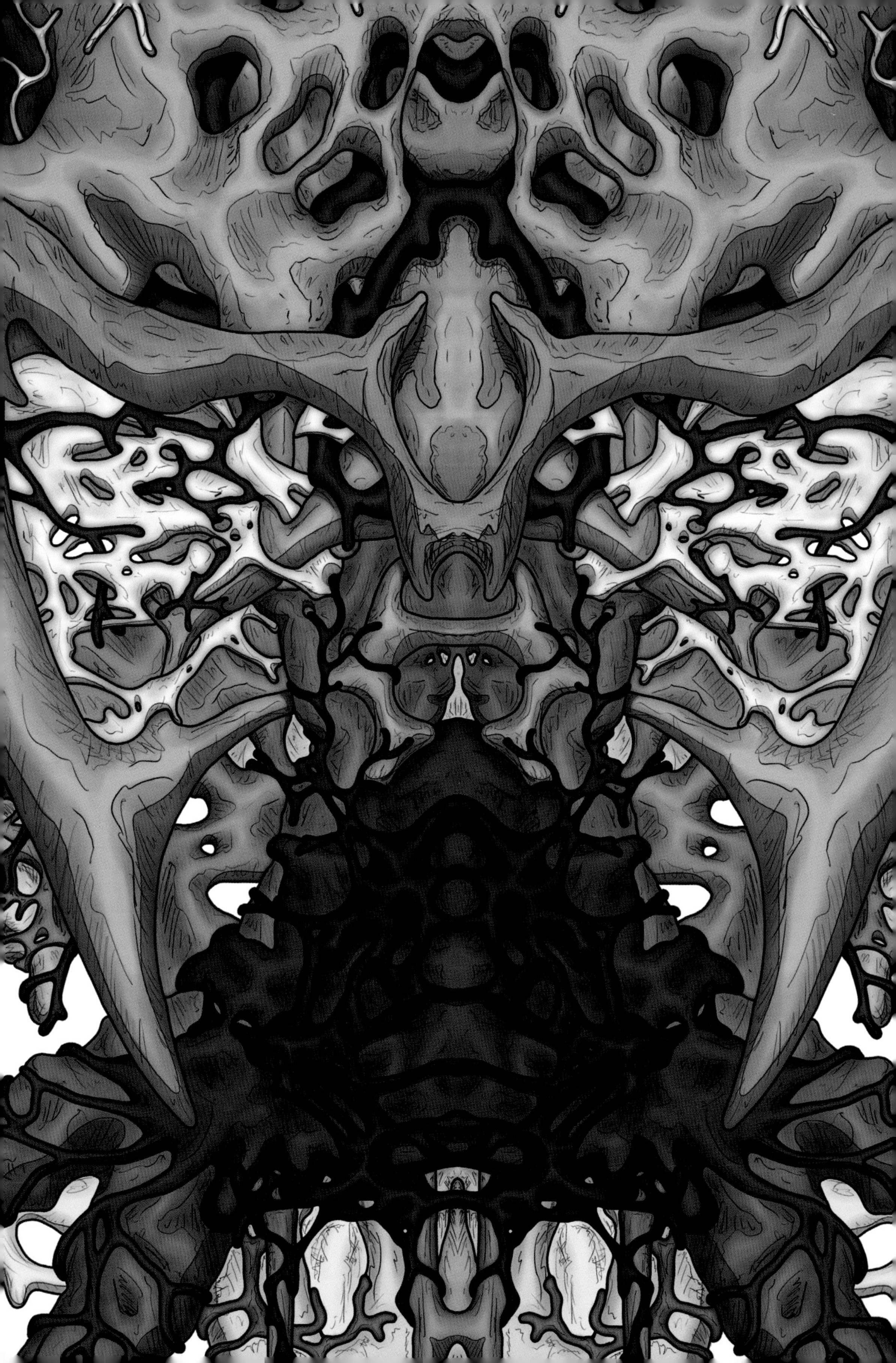

2. Indications for the use of repair tissues

The extended hemilaryngectomy defect

Posterior glottic and subglottic stenosis

Long-segment stenosis and re-stenosis

Tracheal tumor with long-segment involvement

Some laryngeal and tracheal defects cannot be bridged by an end-to-end anastomosis. For these defects, repair tissues will be necessary to reconstruct the defect.

The extended hemilaryngectomy defect

SOME UNILATERAL T2b-T3 GLOTTIC CANCERS WITH SUBGLOTTIC EXTENSION AND LATERALIZED CHONDROSARCOMAS CAN BE REMOVED SAFELY WITH AN EXTENDED PARTIAL LARYNGECTOMY.

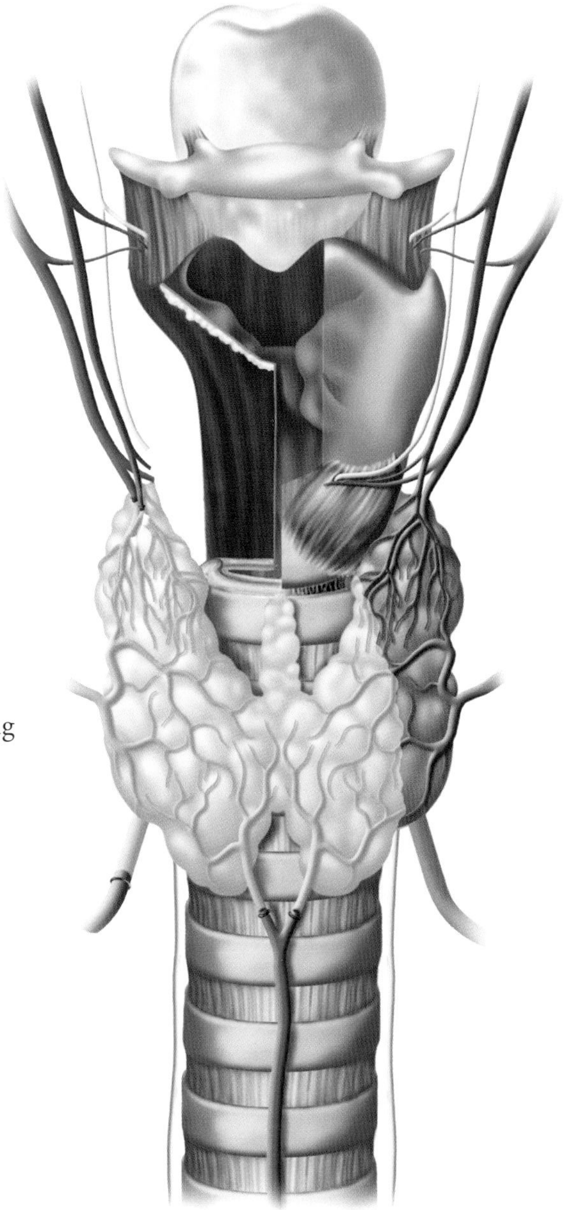

EXTENDED HEMILARYNGECTOMY DEFECT

The resulting glottic-subglottic defect will need tissue reconstruction to preserve all laryngeal functions. The remaining defect after the removal of a significant portion of the cricoid ring results in a collapsed and incompetent upper airway.

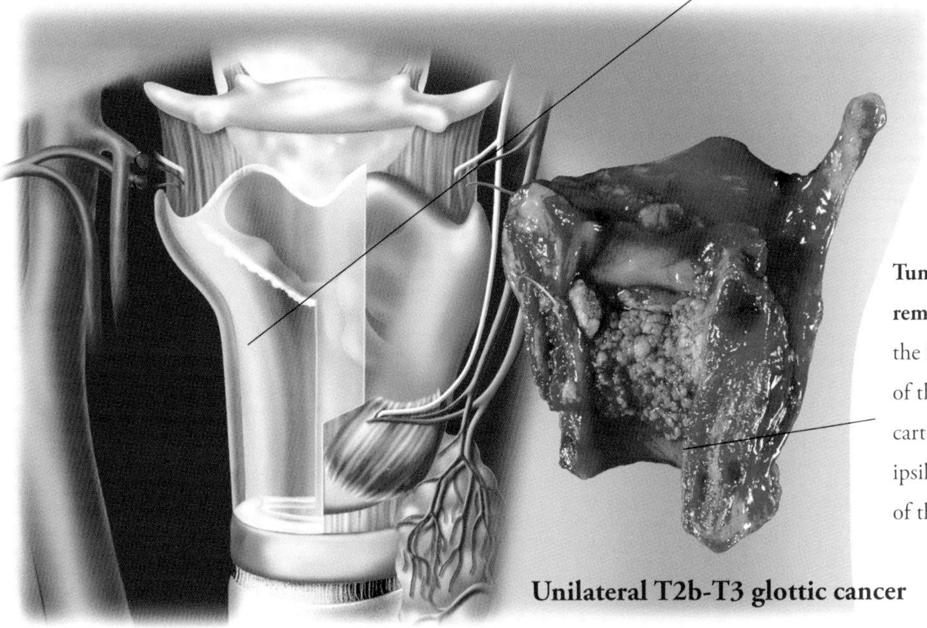
Suitable repair tissue may preserve laryngeal functions and avoid the need for a total laryngectomy.
Tumor removal with the inclusion of the cricoid cartilage on the ipsilateral side of the tumor.

Unilateral T2b-T3 glottic cancer

Coronal view

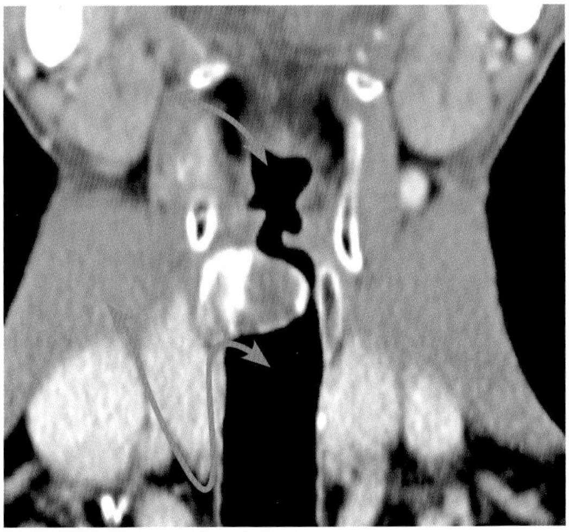

Axial view

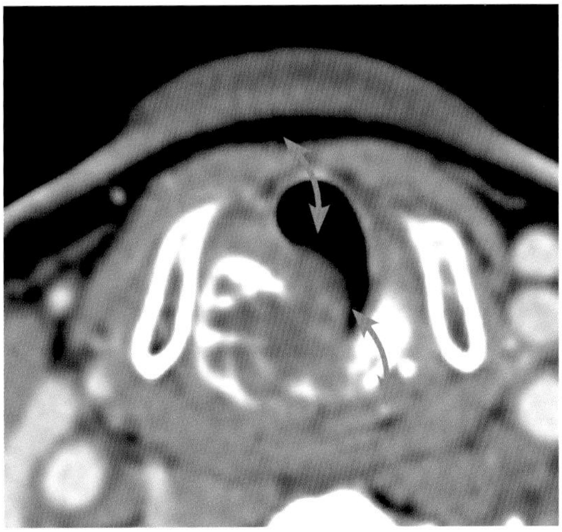

Lateralized chondrosarcoma

Double arrows indicate the extent of the tumor resection.

Posterior glottic and subglottic stenosis

A COMBINED POSTERIOR GLOTTIC AND SUBGLOTTIC STENOSIS WITH POST-INTUBATION ANKYLOSIS OF THE ARYTENOID CARTILAGES CAN BE APPROACHED BY A MIDLINE LARYNGEAL INCISION (FOR GRADE 3 (75%-99%) STENOSIS AND GRADE 4 (NO LUMEN) STENOSIS. THROUGH THE ANTERIOR LARYNGOFISSURE APPROACH, THE POSTERIOR CRICOID IS INCISED AND THE TWO CRICOID HALVES ARE DISTRACTED. REPAIR TISSUE WILL BE NECESSARY TO AUGMENT THE GLOTTIC AND SUBGLOTTIC AIRWAY LUMEN.

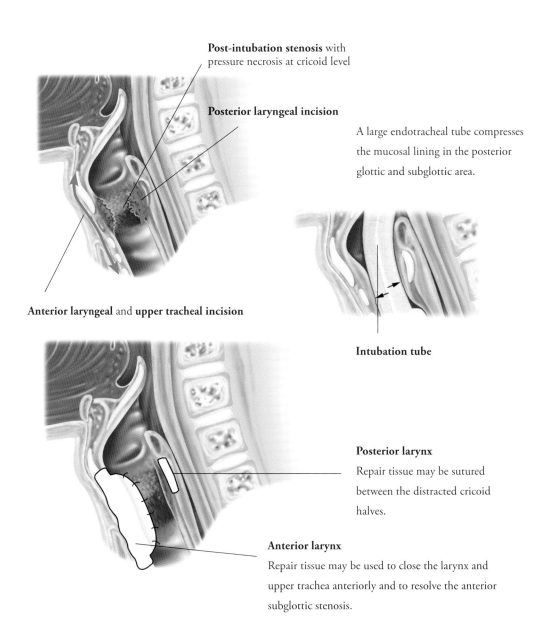

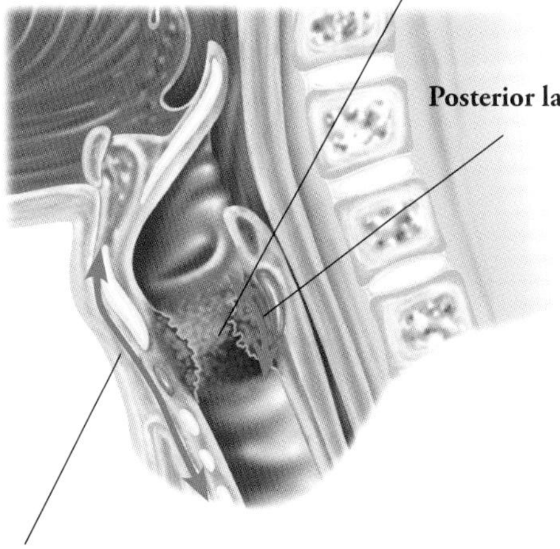
Post-intubation stenosis with pressure necrosis at cricoid level
Posterior laryngeal incision
Anterior laryngeal and **upper tracheal incision**

A large endotracheal tube compresses the mucosal lining in the posterior glottic and subglottic area.

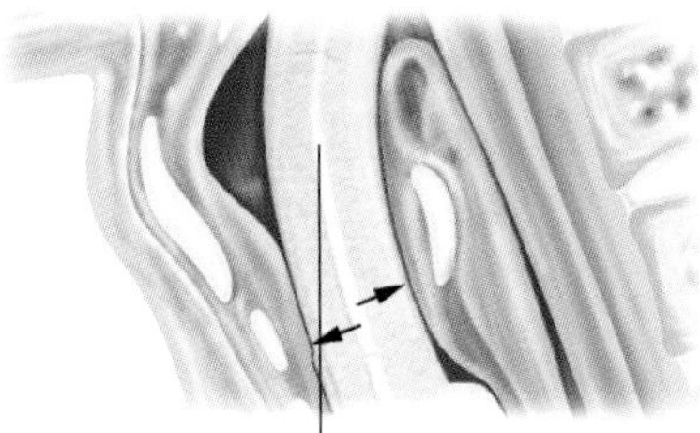
Intubation tube

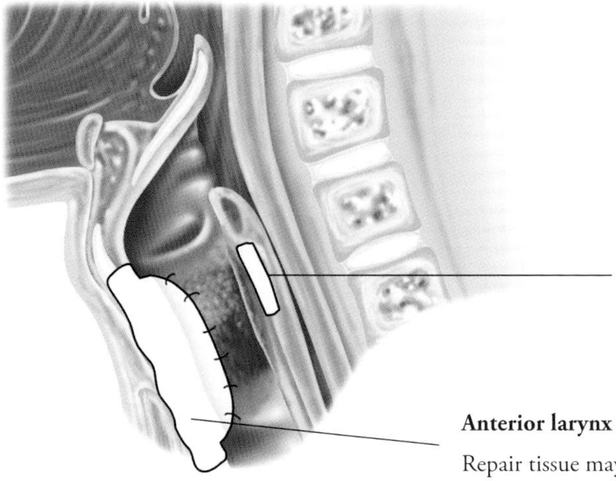
Posterior larynx
Anterior larynx

Posterior larynx
Repair tissue may be sutured between the distracted cricoid halves.

Anterior larynx
Repair tissue may be used to close the larynx and upper trachea anteriorly and to resolve the anterior subglottic stenosis.

Stenosis resulting from secondary healing after pressure necrosis of the mucosal lining

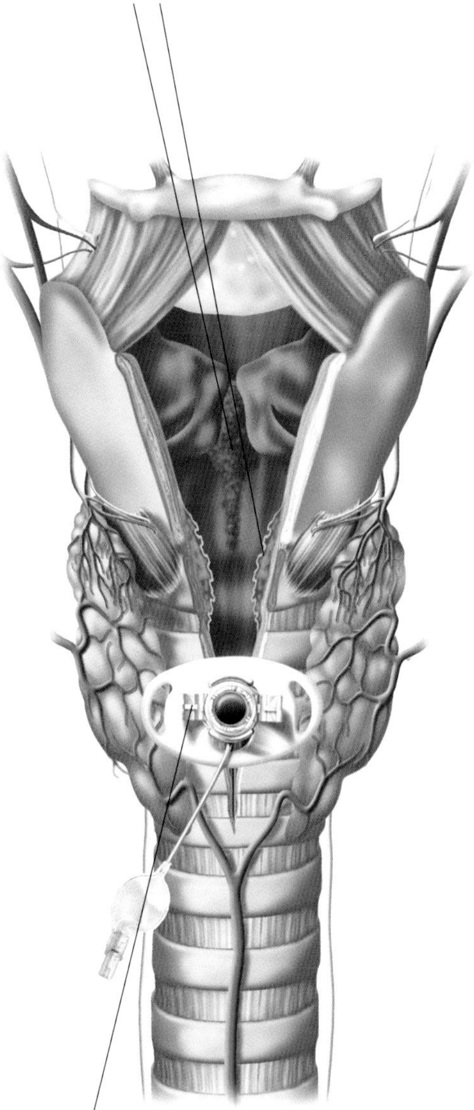

Anterior view after anterior incision

Tracheal cannulation

Repair tissues will be necessary to remove the tracheal cannula and to close the tracheostomy.

Cricoarytenoid joint

Ankylosis of the cricoarytenoid joint

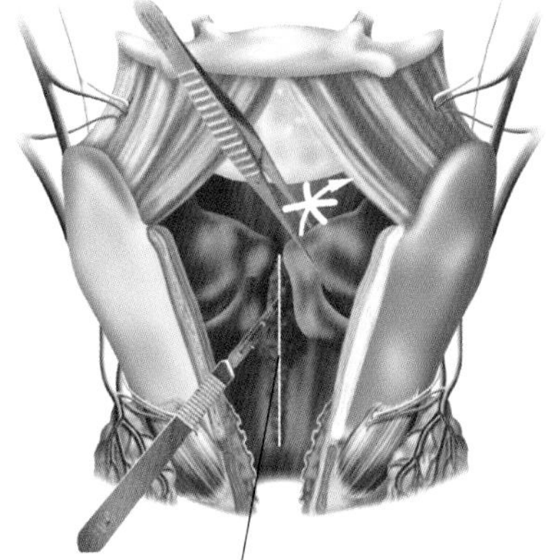

Posterior larynx

Posterior cricoid incision

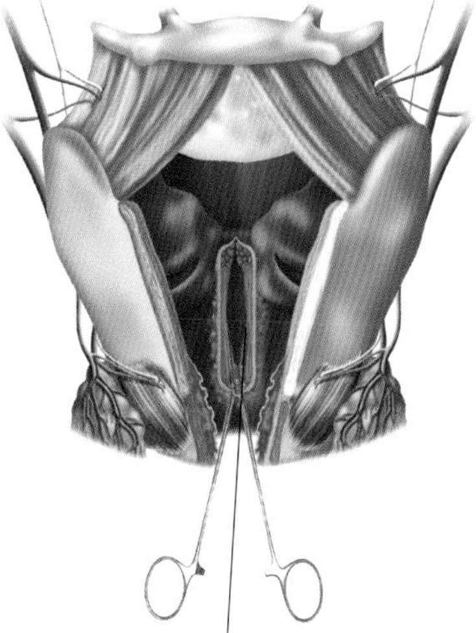

Posterior larynx

Distraction of the posterior incision

Long-segment stenosis and re-stenosis

A LONG-SEGMENT STENOSIS AND A RE-STENOSIS AFTER SEGMENTAL RESECTION CAN BE INCISED ANTERIORLY. AFTER A LONGITUDINAL INCISION, THE STENOTIC SEGMENT IS EXPANDED. REPAIR TISSUE THAT IS PLACED IN THE ANTERIOR DEFECT CAN BE CONSIDERED TO AUGMENT THE AIRWAY LUMEN. AFTER THE INCISION AND EXPANSION OF THESE STENOSES, TWO DIFFERENT SITUATIONS MAY BE ENCOUNTERED: THE INCISED AND EXPANDED NATIVE AIRWAY MAY PRESERVE SUFFICIENT CONCAVITY TO ALLOW FOR A LINEAR RECONSTRUCTION ANTERIORLY OR THE RECONSTRUCTED TISSUE NEEDS TO BUILD A CONVEX-SHAPED RECONSTRUCTION.

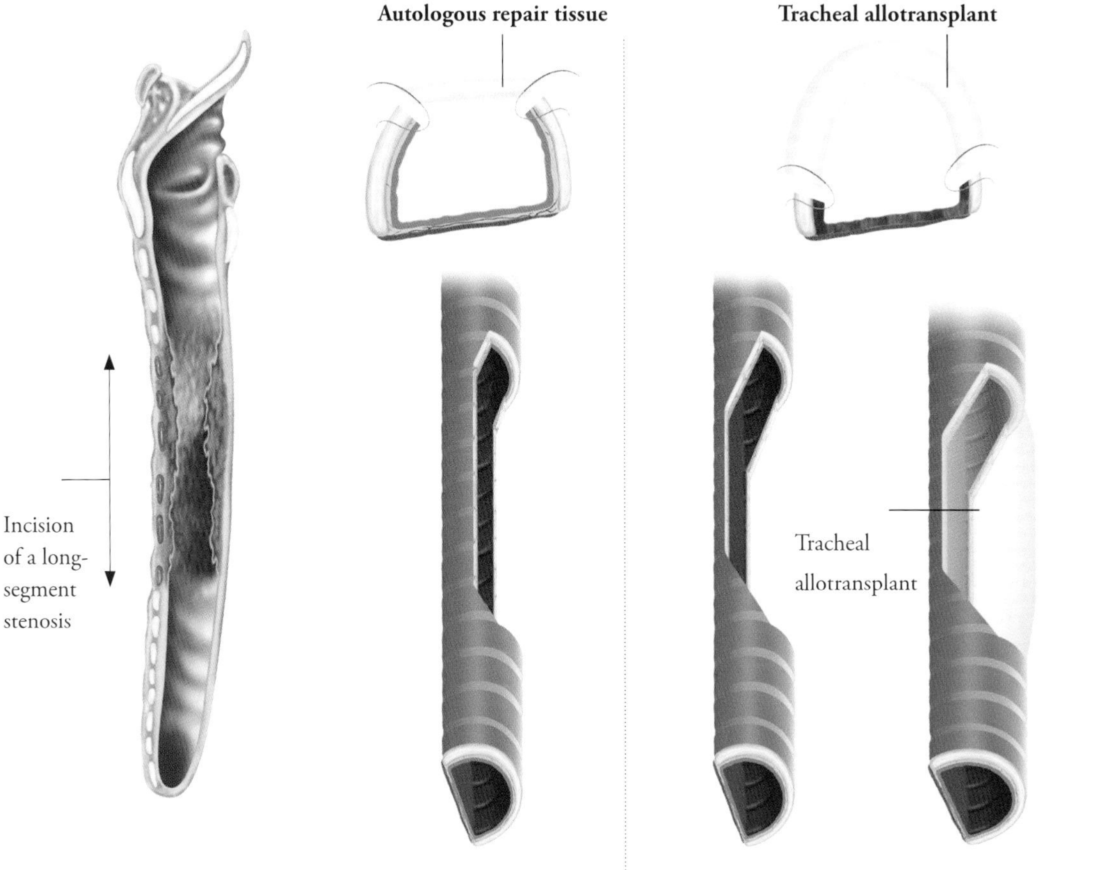
Autologous repair tissue
Tracheal allotransplant
Incision of a long-segment stenosis
Tracheal allotransplant

LINEAR RECONSTRUCTION

Autologous tissue may repair an airway defect linearly. After the incision and expansion of the stenosis, there is sufficient remaining concavity to allow for a linear reconstruction.

CONVEX-SHAPED RECONSTRUCTION

A patch tracheal allotransplant will be necessary to restore the airway lumen. The remaining native airway concavity is not sufficient for a linear reconstruction.

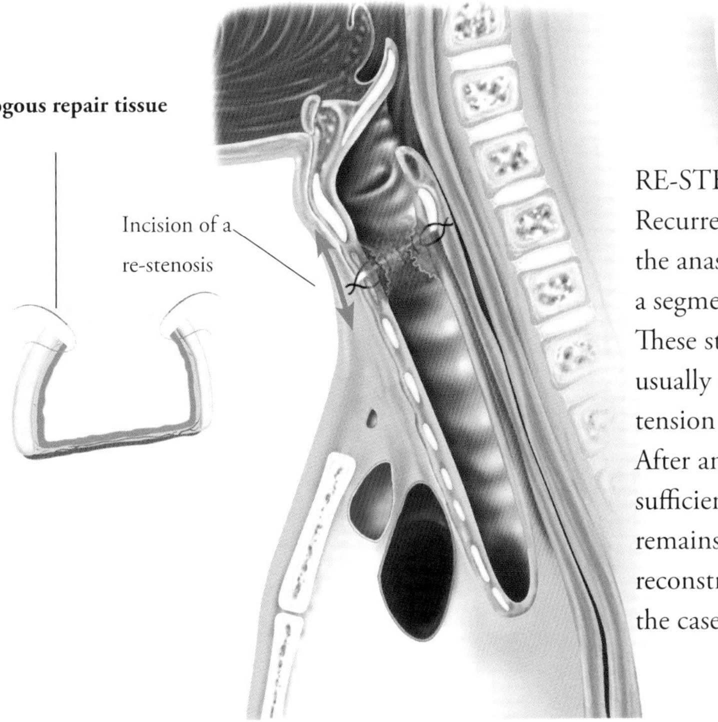
Autologous repair tissue
Incision of a re-stenosis

RE-STENOSIS

Recurrent stenosis at the anastomosis after a segmental resection. These strictures are usually related to excessive tension at the suture line. After anterior incision, sufficient concavity remains to enable a linear reconstruction in most of the cases.

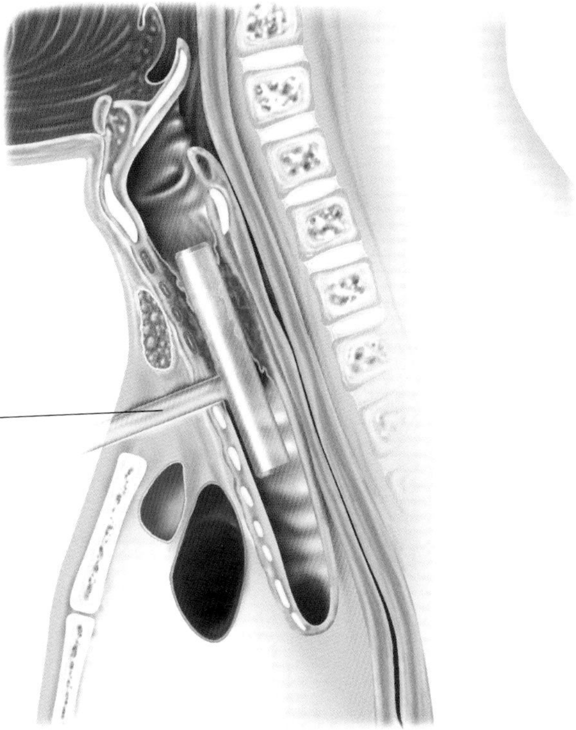

T-tube

A T-tube (or a combination of a stent with a cannula) can be placed through the stenosis as a temporary treatment option.

Tracheal tumor with long-segment involvement

PRIMARY MALIGNANT TRACHEAL TUMORS ARE RARE, ACCOUNTING FOR ONLY 0.2 % OF ALL MALIGNANCIES OF THE RESPIRATORY TRACT. LONG-SEGMENT TUMORAL INVOLVEMENT NECESSITATES TUMOR REMOVAL WITH LONG-SEGMENT TRACHEAL RESECTION.

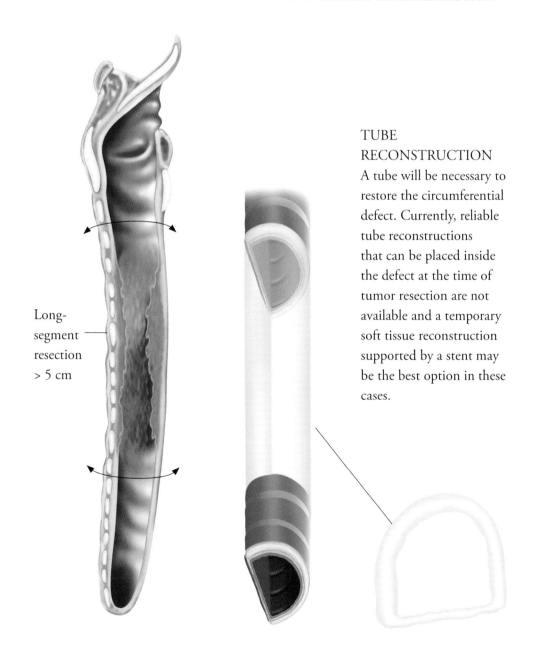

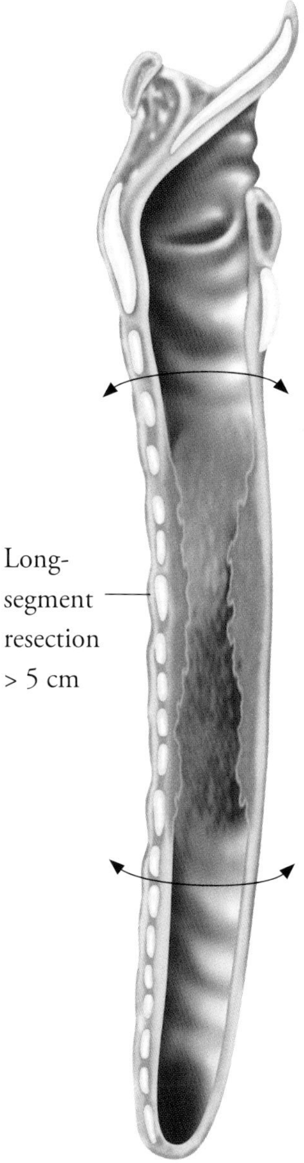
Long-
segment
resection
> 5 cm

TUBE RECONSTRUCTION
A tube will be necessary to restore the circumferential defect. Currently, reliable tube reconstructions that can be placed inside the defect at the time of tumor resection are not available and a temporary soft tissue reconstruction supported by a stent may be the best option in these cases.

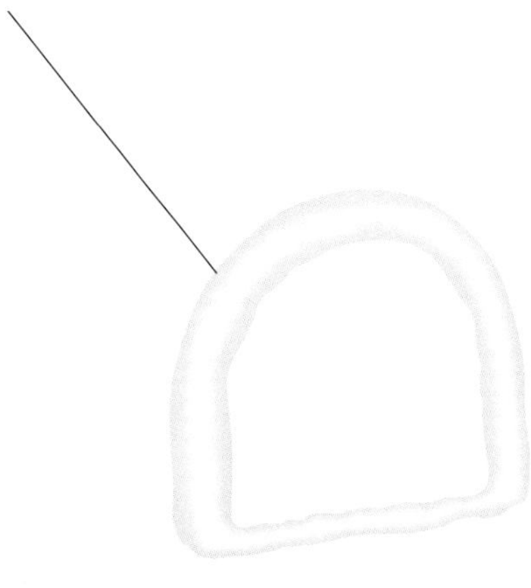

THE CIRCUMFERENTIAL DEFECT

A circumferential defect can be reconstructed temporarily with a stent wrapped in vascularized tissue, such as transposed omentum, or a pedicled or free flap. Wound contraction with shortening of the defect (secondary healing) can be observed for soft tissue reconstructions without epithelial lining (omentum and muscle flaps) and for the aortic graft wrapped with vascularized omentum. This type of reconstruction has to be considered as tempory because of the stent-related complications.

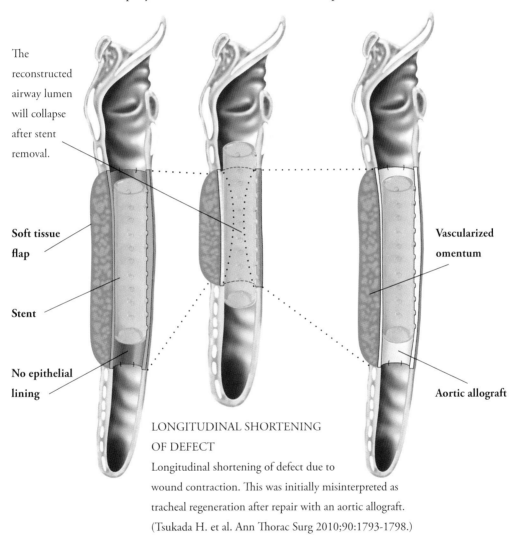

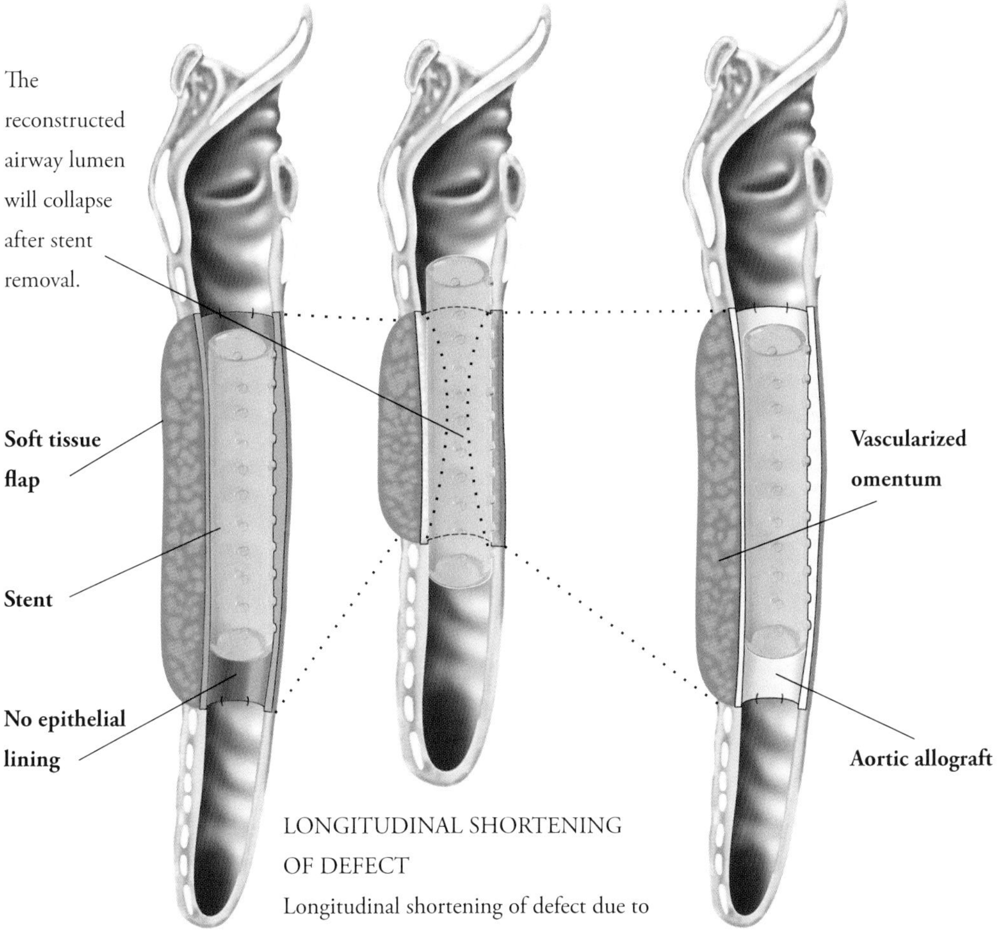
The reconstructed airway lumen will collapse after stent removal.
Soft tissue flap
Stent
No epithelial lining
Vascularized omentum
Aortic allograft

LONGITUDINAL SHORTENING OF DEFECT

Longitudinal shortening of defect due to wound contraction. This was initially misinterpreted as tracheal regeneration after repair with an aortic allograft. (Tsukada H. et al. Ann Thorac Surg 2010;90:1793-1798.)

STENT COMPLICATIONS

- Stent obstruction due to accumulation of secretions.
- Stent migration.
- Granulation tissue formation at the upper and lower end of the stent.
- Halitosis (stent colonization).

UARKIORZ transforms the trachea into several tubes that consist of cartilage rings, embedded in vascular, capillary networks. A remarkable aspect of this design is its graphical, almost tactile qualities, something which one would rather expect from comics or woodcuts.

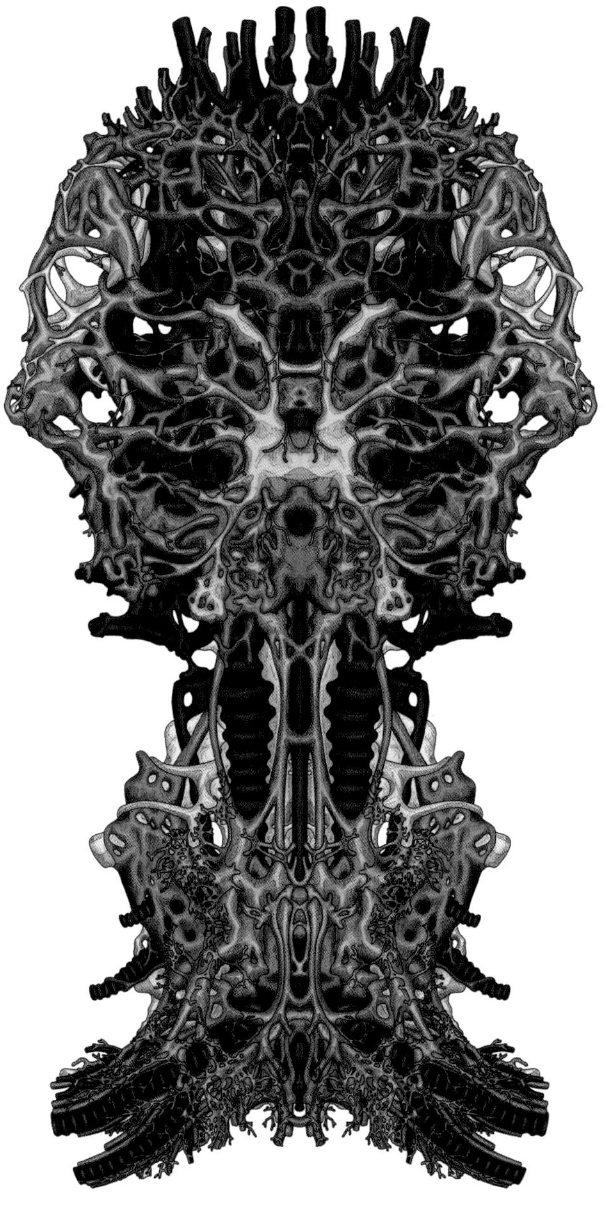

UARKIORZ, 2010-2011

PRINT

155 × 120 CM

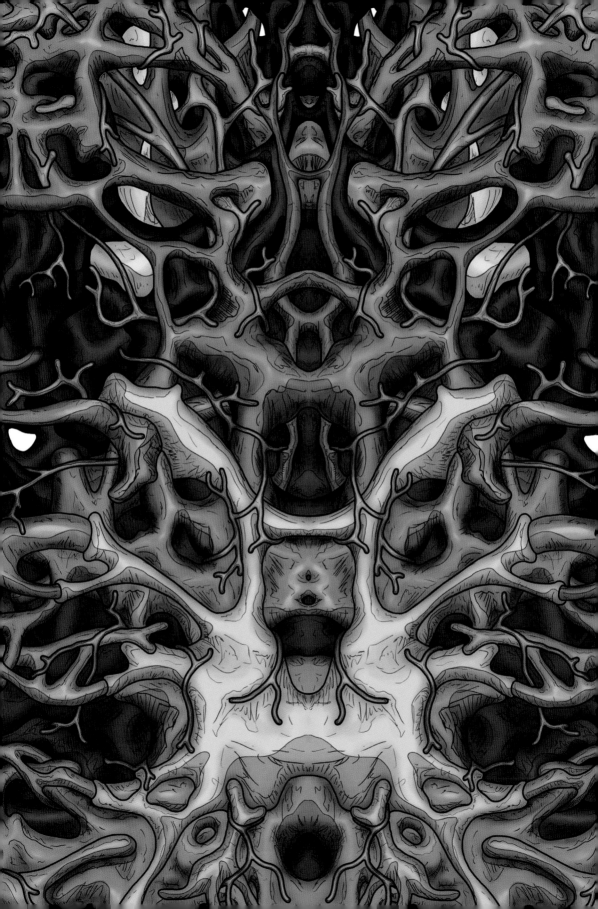

3. Experimental reconstruction

Experimental tracheal revascularization

Inverted autotransplantation and mucociliary clearance

Tracheal autotransplantation and the definition
of an optimal airway repair

Vascularized cartilage grafts – design (1) - (2)

Vascularized cartilage grafts – histology

Secondary healing – design

Secondary healing – histology

Mucosal-lined reconstruction

A rabbit model was developed that enabled for the study of basic airway wound healing mechanisms. The concepts of a mucosa-lined reconstruction, tracheal autotransplantation and tracheal allotransplantation were created with this model.

Experimental tracheal revascularization

ORTHOTOPIC REVASCULARIZATION AND TRACHEAL AUTOTRANSPLANTATION WAS STUDIED IN A RABBIT MODEL.

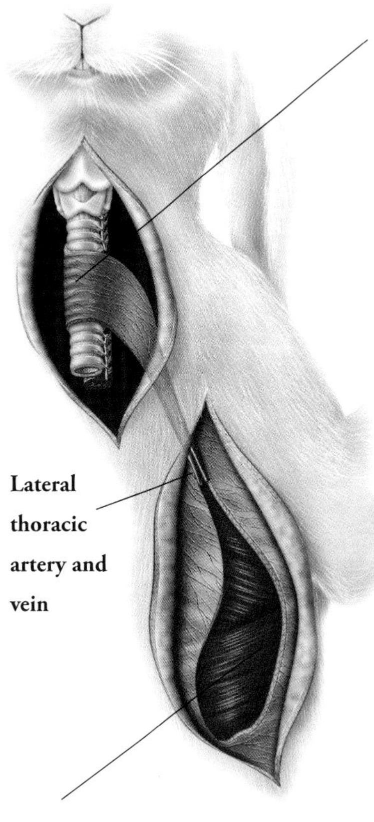
Lateral thoracic artery and vein

ORTHOTOPIC REVASCULARIZATION

The cervical trachea was dissected over 2 cm from the underlying esophagus with disruption of the extrinsic blood supply. The cervical trachea was then wrapped with a transposed lateral thoracic fascial flap. The trachea was not incised, in order that the intrinsic mucosal blood supply was preserved.

LATERAL THORACIC FASCIAL FLAP

The lateral thoracic fascial flap is situated subcutaneously on the lateral chest wall. This thin, subcutaneous tissue and fascial flap is supplied by the lateral thoracic vessels that emerge from axillary vessels. The flap can be rotated into the neck region with the preservation of the vascular pedicle.

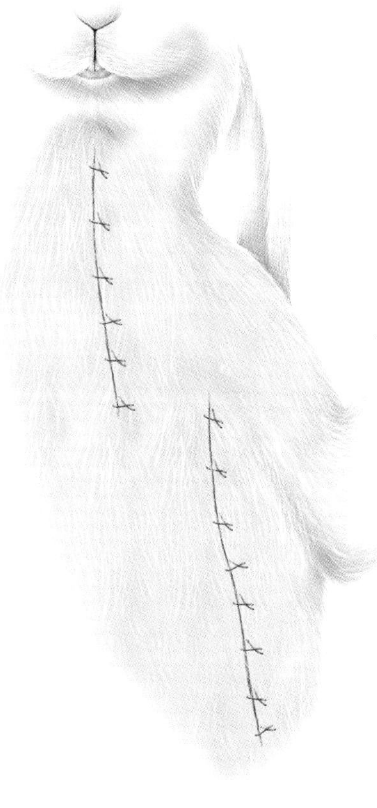

SKIN CLOSURE

The skin incisions were closed and the fascial flap-enwrapped segment became revascularized in the orthotopic position. A moderately ischemic trachea is beneficial for the induction of revascularization by the lateral thoracic fascial flap. The preserved intrinsic tracheal blood supply means that revascularization can occur without the risk of avascular necrosis.

MACROSCOPY
After the posterior longitudinal incision of the trachea, the mucosal lining revealed a 2-cm segment of trachea that was intensely stained by blue silicone.

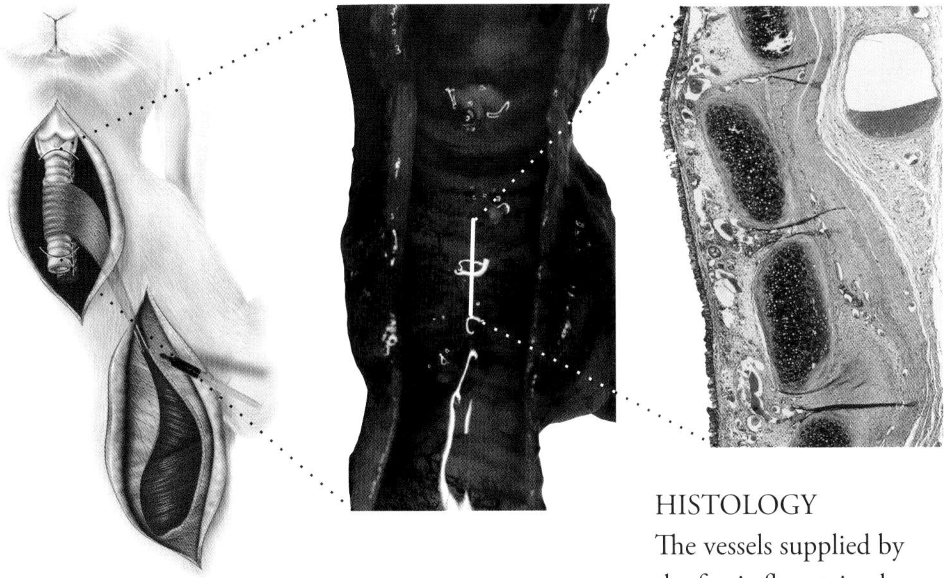

AFTER 14 DAYS
The amount of tracheal revascularization was visualized after the injection of blue silicone into the fascial flap artery.

HISTOLOGY
The vessels supplied by the fascia flap stained blue. Revascularization occurred by 'vascular induction' through the intercartilaginous ligaments.

> "Cartilaginous tissue does not allow for the ingrowth of blood vessels. Vascular connections between the flap and submucosal space occur at the intercartilaginous ligaments."

Inverted autotransplantation and mucociliary clearance

THE TECHNIQUE OF ORTHOTOPIC TRACHEAL REVASCULARIZATION COULD BE USED TO EXAMINE THE MUCOCILIARY CLEARANCE FOLLOWING SEGMENTAL TRACHEAL AUTOTRANSPLANTATION IN THE REVERSED POSITION. THESE INVERSELY TRANSPLANTED TRACHEAS SHOWED THAT BOTH THE MUCOCILIARY ORIENTATION AND COORDINATION FULLY RECOVERED. HOWEVER, SURGICAL REVERSAL OF A TRACHEAL SEGMENT DID NOT REPROGRAM THE POLARITY OF THE CILIA, WHICH INDICATED THAT THIS POLARITY WAS NOT INFLUENCED BY EXTERNAL FACTORS SUCH AS AIRFLOW AND MUCUS FLOW IN THE TRACHEAL LUMEN.

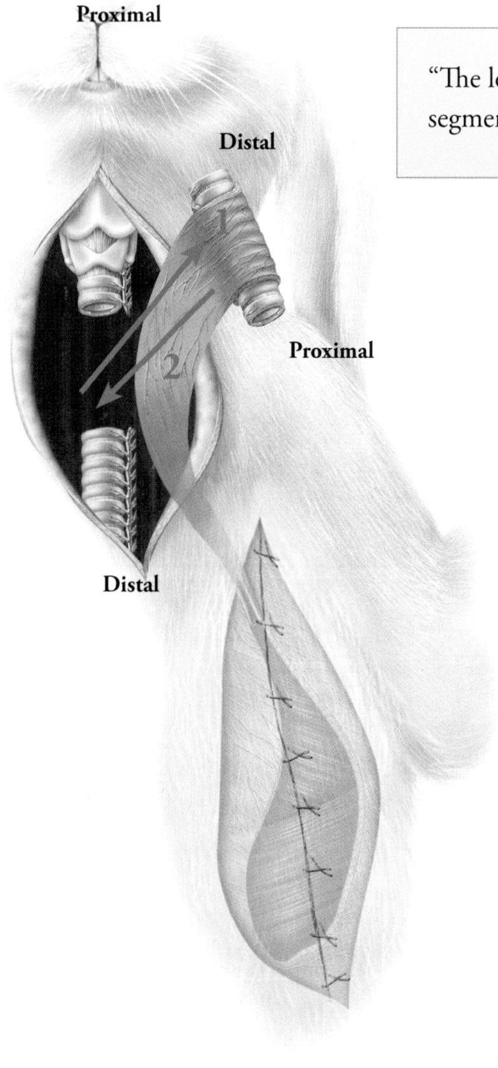
Proximal
Distal
1
2
Proximal
Distal

"The loss of mucociliary clearance over a reconstructed segment of the trachea can be cleared by coughing."

REVERSED TRACHEAL AUTOTRANSPLANTATION

A 2-cm segment of trachea was excised and reversed 2 weeks after orthotopic revascularization (1). After reversal, the segment was re-introduced into the airway tract (2).

Mucociliary clearance was examined one month after the re-implantation of the reserved segment. After the posterior longitudinal incision of the laryngotracheal complex, the movement of silicone particles was evaluated immediately post-mortem, when the trachea was pinned onto a vertically placed cardboard.

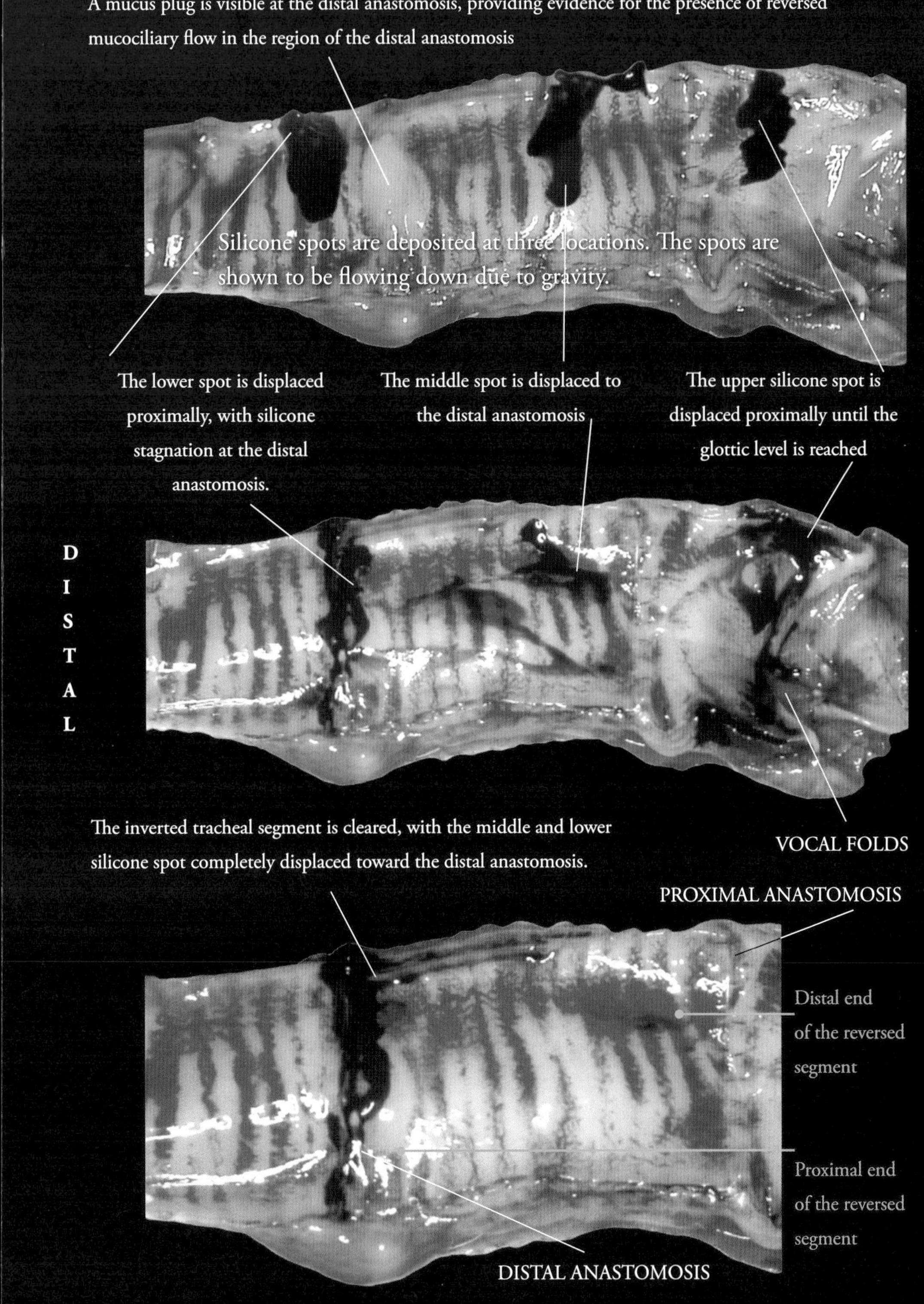
A mucus plug is visible at the distal anastomosis, providing evidence for the presence of reversed mucociliary flow in the region of the distal anastomosis
Silicone spots are deposited at three locations. The spots are shown to be flowing down due to gravity.
The lower spot is displaced proximally, with silicone stagnation at the distal anastomosis.
The middle spot is displaced to the distal anastomosis
The upper silicone spot is displaced proximally until the glottic level is reached
D I S T A L
VOCAL FOLDS
The inverted tracheal segment is cleared, with the middle and lower silicone spot completely displaced toward the distal anastomosis.
PROXIMAL ANASTOMOSIS
Distal end of the reversed segment
Proximal end of the reversed segment
DISTAL ANASTOMOSIS

POSTMORTEM MUCOCILIARY CLEARANCE ON THE EXCISED LARYNGOTRACHEAL COMPLEX ONE MONTH AFTER RE-IMPLANTATION

Tracheal autotransplantation and the definition of an optimal airway repair

THE CONCEPT OF ORTHOTOPICAL REVASCULARIZATION OF A TRACHEAL SEGMENT CAN BE USED TO RECONSTRUCT EXTENDED HEMILARYNGECTOMY DEFECTS DURING TRACHEAL AUTOTRANSPLANTATION.

SEGMENTAL BLOOD SUPPLY OF THE CERVICAL TRACHEA

The typical arterial blood supply, consisting of several tracheo-esophageal branches originating from the inferior thyroid artery and venous drainage of the trachea do not enable direct, microvascular reperfusion.

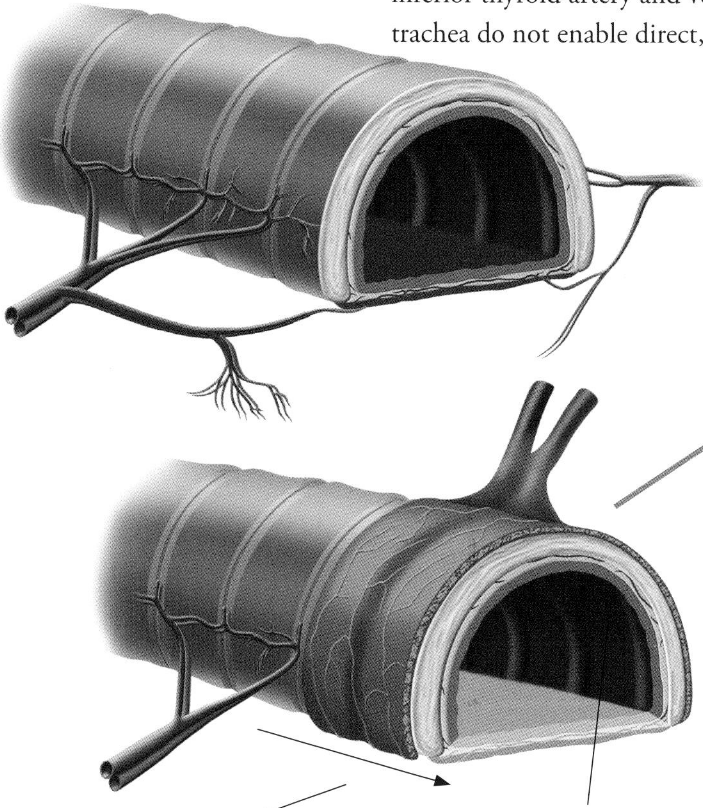

Experimental tracheal autotransplantation of an extende hemilaryngectomy defect

ORTHOTOPICAL REVASCULARIZATION

A thin, vascularized fascial flap supplies the cartilaginous trachea. The vascular pedicle of the fascial flap allows for the transfer of the revascularized trachea **two weeks after** orthotopical revascularization.

Tracheal continuity can be restored by bringing up the remaining trachea to the reconstructed larynx.

OPTIMAL REPAIR TISSUE

The optimal tissue for reconstruction is provided by a segment of cartilaginous trachea with three typical characteristics: blood supply, mucosal lining and cartilaginous support.

EXPERIMENTAL TRACHEAL AUTOTRANSPLANT USED FOR HEMILARYNX RECONSTRUCTION (ONE MONTH AFTER AUTOTRANSPLANTATION)

GLOTTIC LEVEL

Native larynx

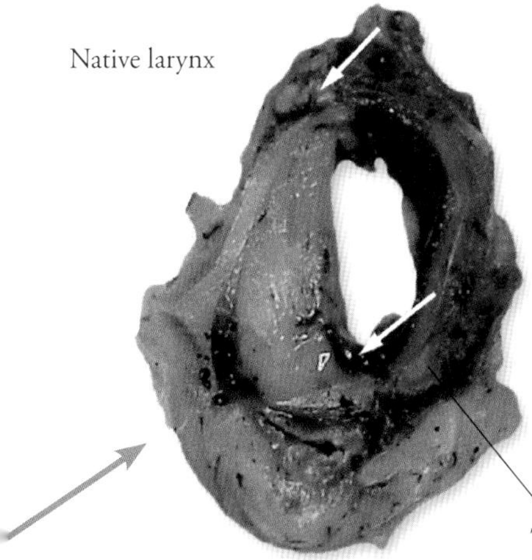

Native larynx

Less convexity at the glottic level

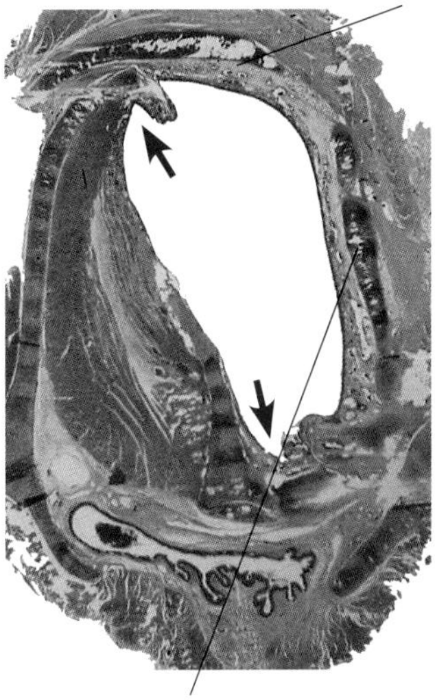

TRACHEAL AUTORANSPLANT

A tracheal autotransplant (between arrows) was used for hemilarynx reconstruction. The artery of the fascial flap was injected with blue silicone.

SUBGLOTTIC LEVEL

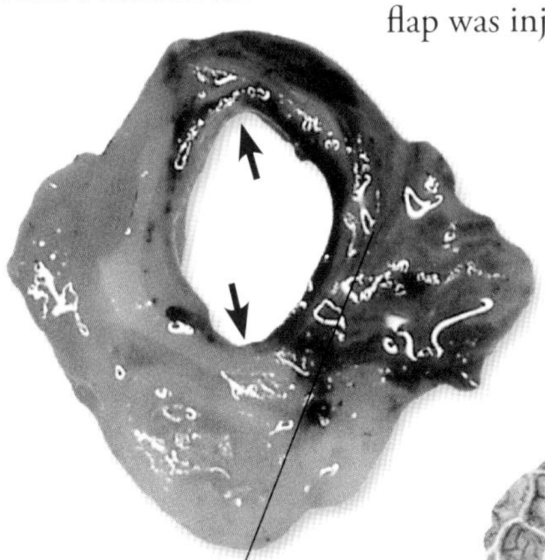

More convexity
at the subglottic level

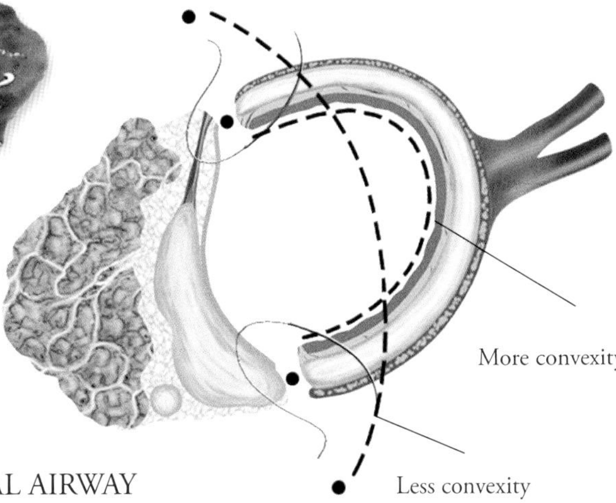

More convexity

Less convexity

DEFINITION OF 'THE OPTIMAL AIRWAY SUPPORT' PROVIDED BY REPAIR TISSUE

The extent of external airway support provided by the reconstructive tissue is shown by the dotted lines. The same tracheal transplant will provide more or less convexity, depending on the width of the defect.

Vascularized cartilage grafts – design (1)

THE IMPORTANCE OF THE MUCOSAL LINING IN AIRWAY REPAIR CAN BE STUDIED WITH VASCULARIZED TUBES OF CARTILAGE. THE HEALING OF A VASCULARIZED CARTILAGINOUS TUBE CAN BE STUDIED EXPERIMENTALLY IN RABBITS. THREE OPERATIONS ARE NECESSARY.

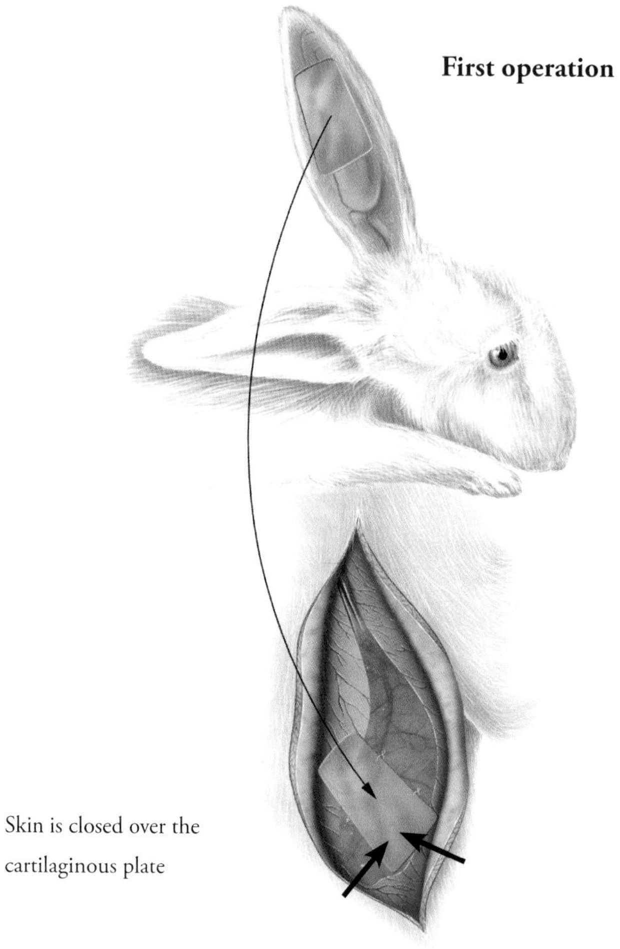
First operation
Skin is closed over the cartilaginous plate

AUTOTRANSPLANTATION OF CARTILAGE

A segment of ear cartilage (20 x 20 mm) is transferred to the lateral thoracic fascia (long arrow). The fascia is then sutured to one side of the cartilaginous patch and the skin is closed (thick arrows) over the cartilage.

Second operation after 2 weeks

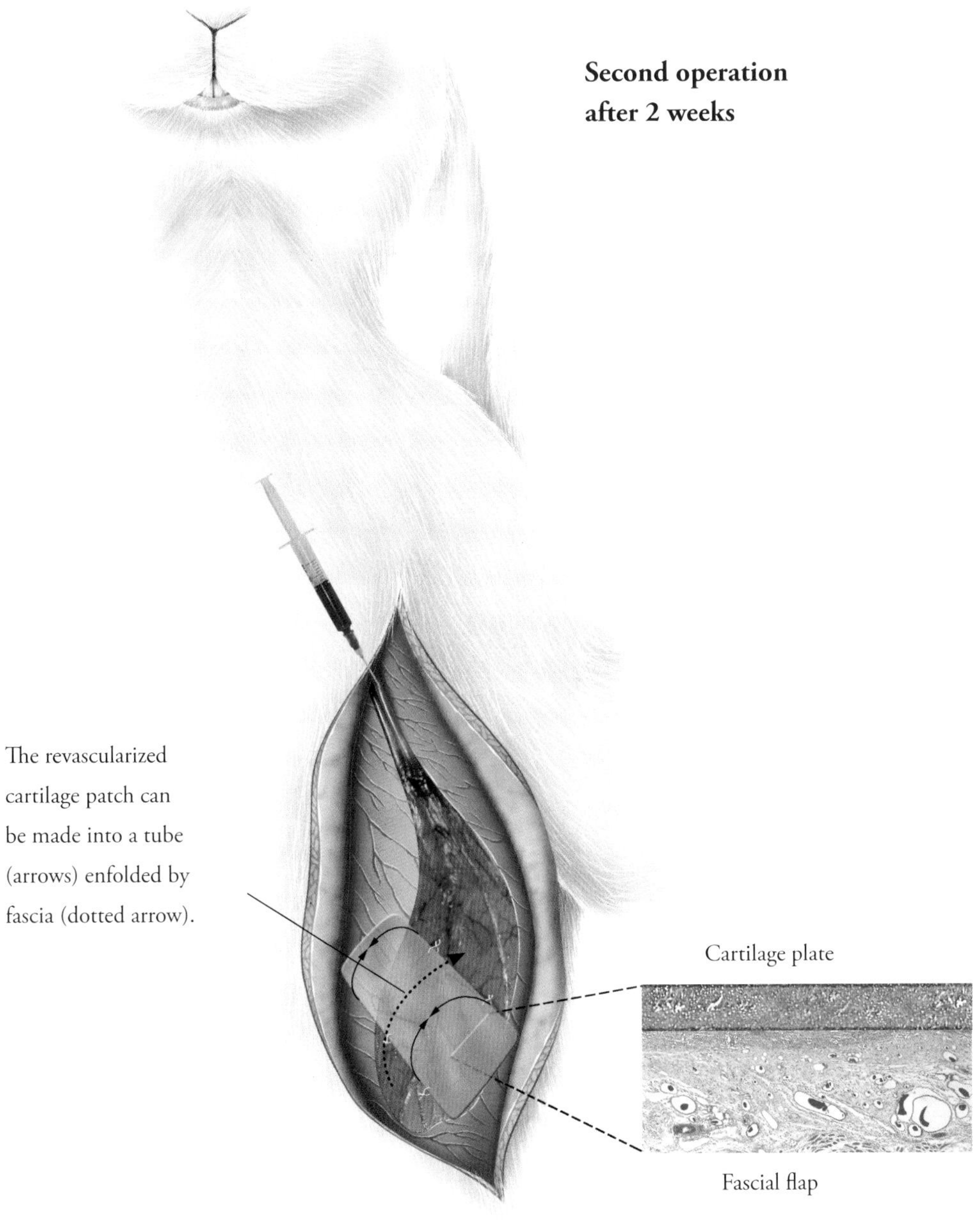
The revascularized cartilage patch can be made into a tube (arrows) enfolded by fascia (dotted arrow).
Cartilage plate
Fascial flap

REVASCULARIZED CARTILAGE

After 14 days, the cartilaginous plate is extensively connected to the fascia. The histological findings after a blue silicone injection show viable cartilage connected to the silicone-injected fascia. The patch can then be made into a tube.

Vascularized cartilage grafts – design (2)

HEALING OF A VASCULARIZED CARTILAGINOUS TUBE CAN BE STUDIED EXPERIMENTALLY IN RABBITS WITH A TRACHEAL REPLACEMENT CONSISTING OF A 2-CM LENGTH TUBE. IN HUMANS, IT MAY BECOME POSSIBLE IN THE FUTURE TO PRODUCE SIMILAR TUBES OF CARTILAGE WITH TISSUE ENGINEERING TECHNIQUES.

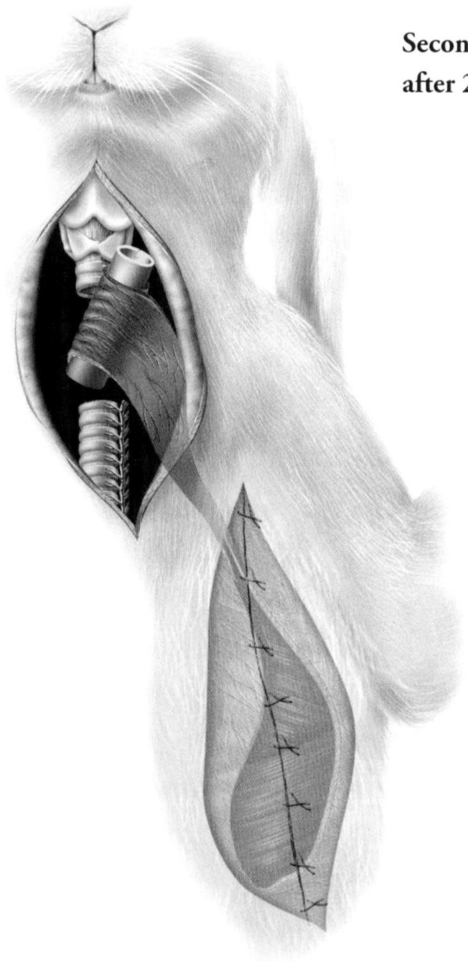

Second operation after 2 weeks

VASCULARIZED CARTILAGE TUBE FOR AIRWAY REPAIR

After 2 weeks, the cartilage patch is made into a 'fascial flap-wrapped tube' with a 2-cm length. A 2-cm segment of the cervical trachea is then removed and the revascularized cartilaginous tube can be sutured into the airway defect.

Third operation after 6 weeks (4 weeks of healing inside the airway tract)

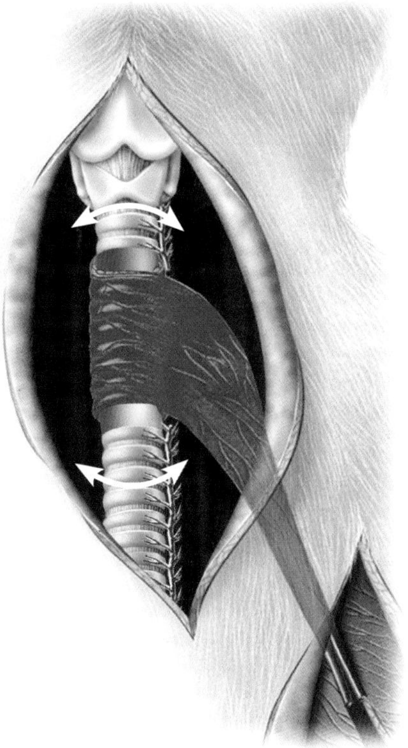

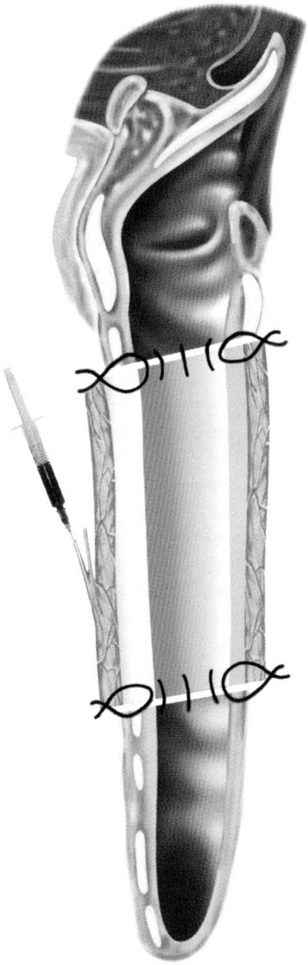

HARVEST OF THE TRACHEAL REPAIR

Rabbits with a tracheal replacement that consisted of a 2-cm length of vascularized cartilage became dyspneic after 4 weeks of healing inside the airway tract. At that time, the artery of the fascial flap was injected with blue silicone and the reconstructed cervical trachea was excised (double arrows) and opened anteriorly for both macroscopic and histological examinations.

Vascularized cartilage grafts – histology

ANIMALS WITH A VASCULARIZED CARTILAGE TUBE BECAME DYSPNEIC AT 4 WEEKS INTO THE HEALING PERIOD. THIS WAS DUE TO THE INTERNAL SIDE OF THE BARE CARTILAGE IN THE MIDDLE OF THE TUBE BEING ATTACKED BY THE HOSTILE ENVIRONMENT OF THE AIRWAY LUMEN. THIS BARE CARTILAGE UNDERWENT NECROSIS WITH THE LOSS OF AIRWAY SUPPORT.

Macroscopic view after follow-up **Histological findings at the anastomosis**

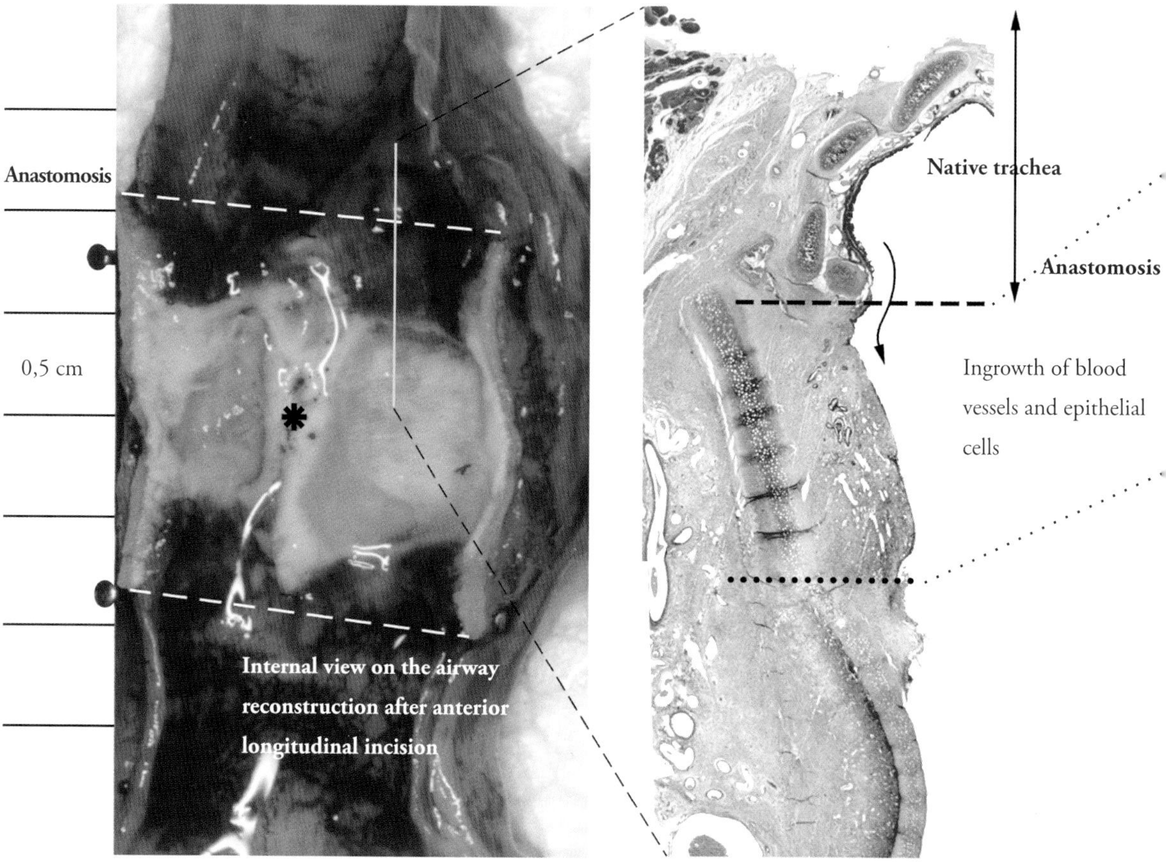
Anastomosis
0,5 cm
*
Internal view on the airway reconstruction after anterior longitudinal incision
Native trachea
Anastomosis
Ingrowth of blood vessels and epithelial cells

POSTMORTEM EVALUATION

White dotted lines indicate the upper and lower anastomosis. An area of approximately 4 mm of the cartilaginous tube is lined with a blue colored mucosal lining at both anastomoses. The middle 1.2 cm of the tube consists of bare cartilage. The posterior suture line is indicated by an asterisk.

HISTOLOGICAL DETAILS (AFTER 4 WEEKS OF HEALING INSIDE THE AIRWAY TRACT)

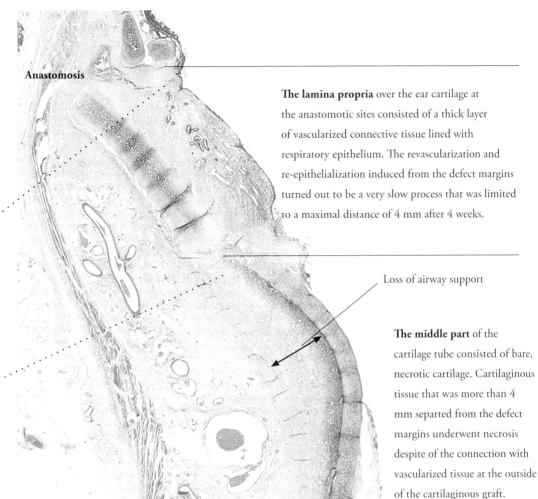

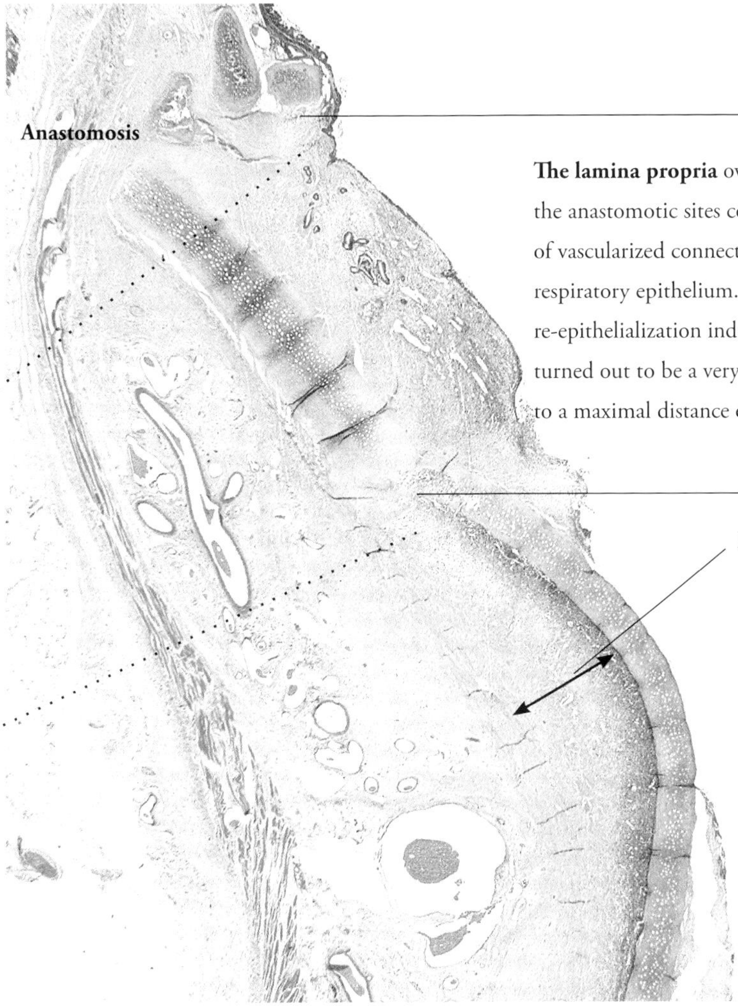
Anastomosis
Loss of airway support

The lamina propria over the ear cartilage at the anastomotic sites consisted of a thick layer of vascularized connective tissue lined with respiratory epithelium. The revascularization and re-epithelialization induced from the defect margins turned out to be a very slow process that was limited to a maximal distance of 4 mm after 4 weeks.

The middle part of the cartilage tube consisted of bare, necrotic cartilage. Cartilaginous tissue that was more than 4 mm separted from the defect margins underwent necrosis despite of the connection with vascularized tissue at the outside of the cartilaginous graft.

"Revascularization and re-epithelialization of the internal site of a vascularized cartilage tube occurs over a short distance at the anastomoses."

"Long-standing airway exposure of bare (vascularized) cartilage leads to necrosis and the loss of support."

"The progress in tracheal reconstruction with engineered cartilage tubes would be modest because of the necessity for obtaining both a blood supply and an epithelial lining at the internal site of the cartilage tube."

Secondary healing – design

FULL-THICKNESS MUCOSAL DEFECTS OF THE AIRWAY WILL HEAL BY SECONDARY INTENTION. FULL-THICKNESS WOUNDS INVOLVE THE REMOVAL OF THE EPITHELIAL LINING AND SUBMUCOSAL SPACE. THE SECONDARY HEALING OF SKIN DEFECTS HAS BEEN STUDIED INTENSIVELY. MUCH LESS IS KNOWN ABOUT MUCOSAL HEALING INSIDE THE AIRWAY BECAUSE OF THE LACK OF RELIABLE

After exteriorization, partial and circumferential full-thickness wounds were made with microscissors.

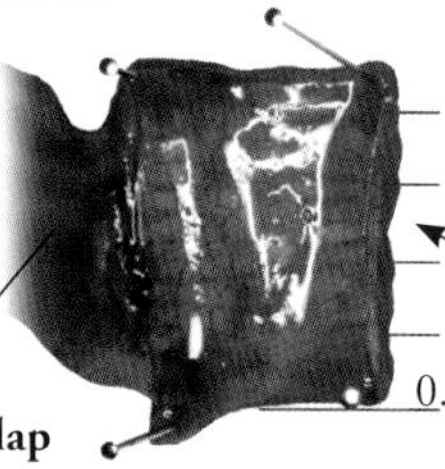
0.5 cm
Fascial flap

After 2 weeks of revascularization

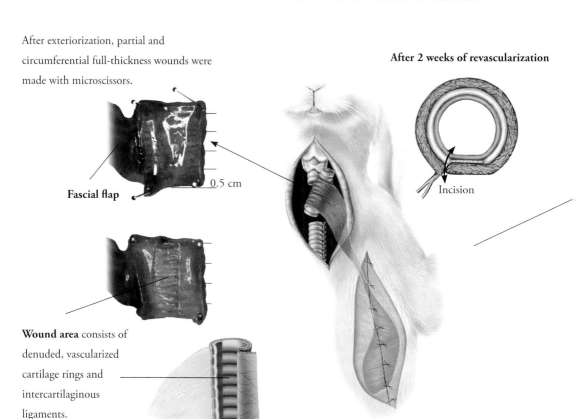

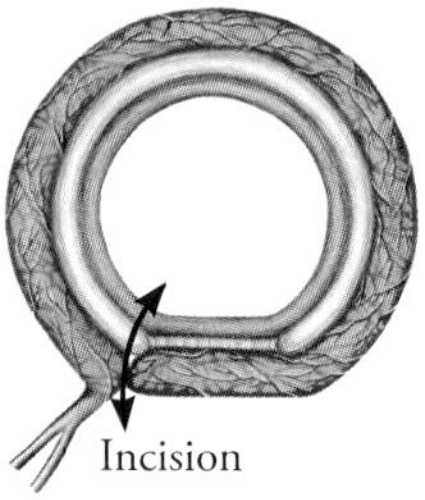
Incision

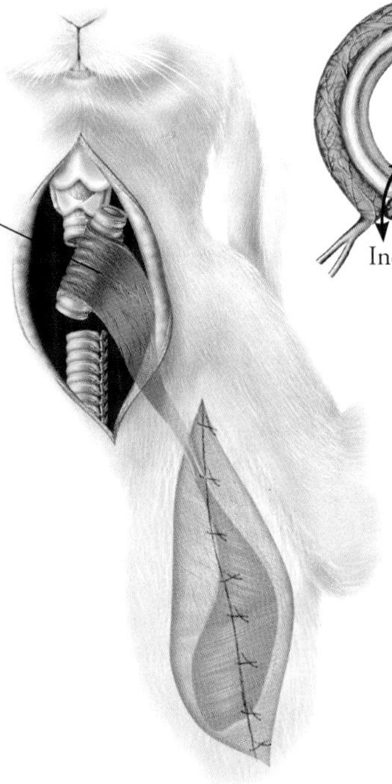

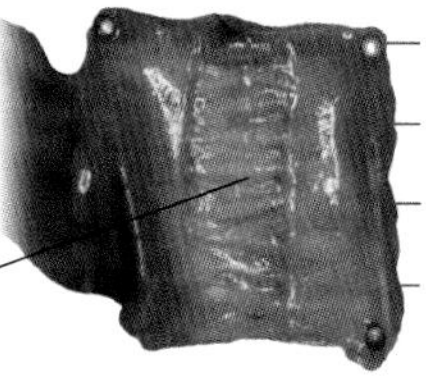

Wound area consists of denuded, vascularized cartilage rings and intercartilaginous ligaments.

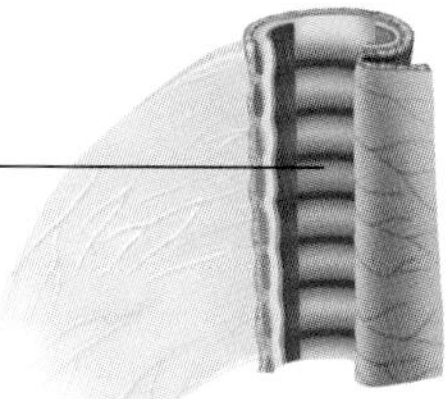

ANTERIOR MUCOSAL DEFECT

An anterior full-thickness mucosal defect that was sharply demarcated from the intact mucosa can be created on the exposed internal site of the tracheal tube.

EXTERIORIZATION OF THE INTERNAL LINING

The fascial-enwrapped tracheal segment is removed from the airway after 2 weeks of orthotopic revascularization. After isolation, the tracheal tube is incised and opened at the membranous trachea. After the full-thickness defect was created, the trachea was closed and reintroduced into the airway tract. Healing was evaluated **4 weeks after re-implantation** into the airway tract.

WOUND HEALING MODELS. AN INVASIVE IN VIVO WOUND HEALING MODEL WAS DEVELOPED WITHOUT INTERFERENTION WITH THE AIRWAY'S BLOOD SUPPLY AND THE AIRWAY'S CARTILAGE SUPPORT. THE MODEL CONSISTS OF A COMPLETE ISOLATION OF TRACHEAL SEGMENTS AFTER PREVIOUS TRACHEAL REVASCULARIZATION. WITH THIS MODEL, THE INTERNAL SITE OF THE TRACHEA WAS EXTERIORIZED AND THE TRACHEA COULD BE REIMPLANTED AFTER WOUNDING.

CIRCUMFERENTIAL FULL-THICKNESS DEFECT

The mucosal lining is completely removed after revascularization and after the isolation of the tracheal segment. Healing was evaluated at the time the animal became dyspneic.

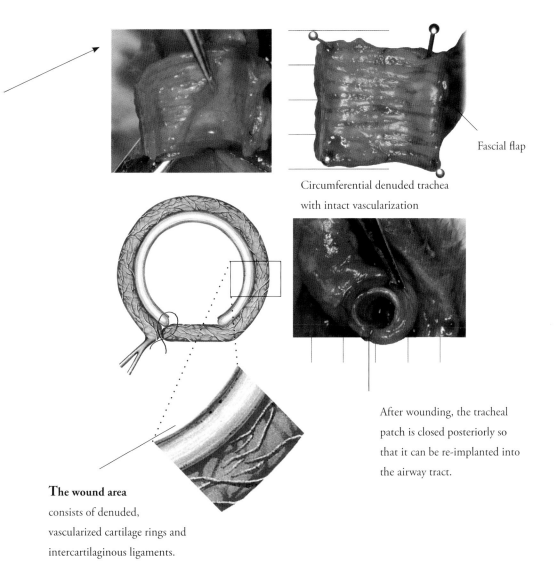

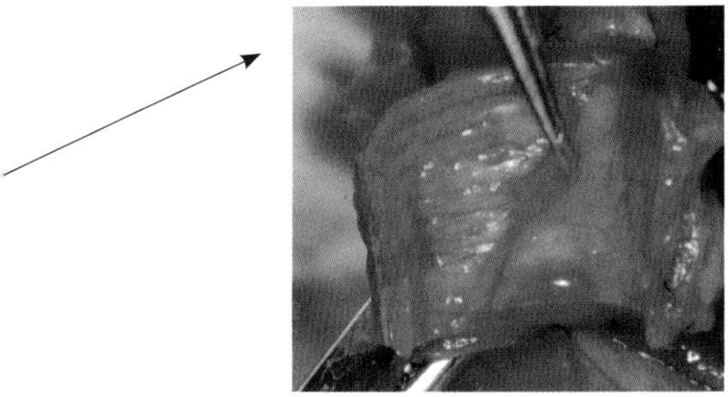

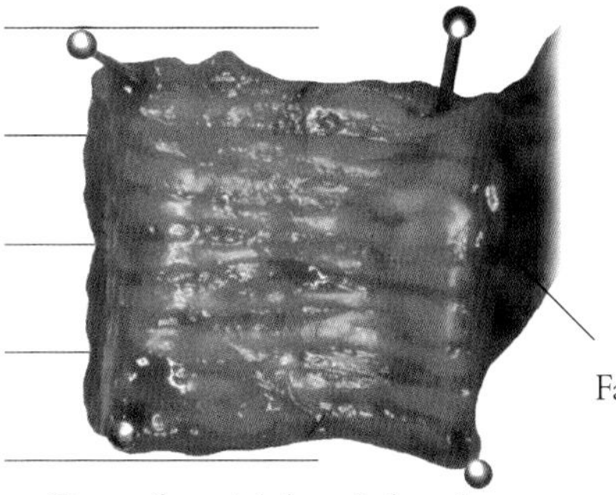
Fascial flap

Circumferential denuded trachea with intact vascularization

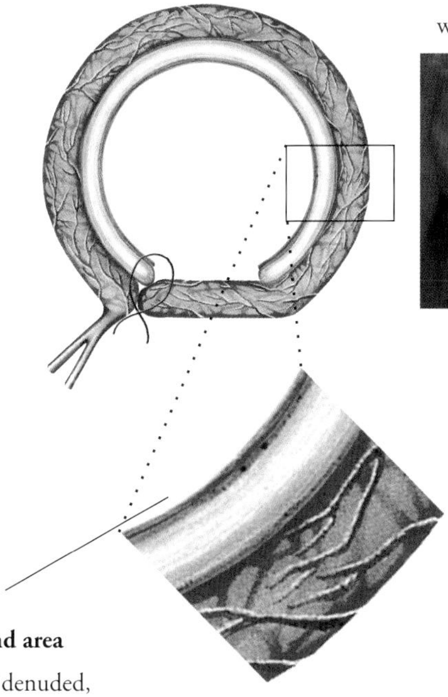

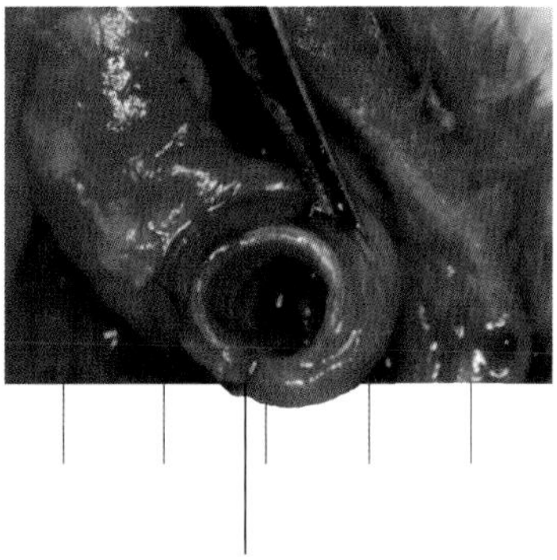

After wounding, the tracheal patch is closed posteriorly so that it can be re-implanted into the airway tract.

The wound area consists of denuded, vascularized cartilage rings and intercartilaginous ligaments.

Secondary healing – histology

ANIMALS WITH A PARTIAL, ANTERIOR WOUND REMAINED WITHOUT SYMPTOMS AND THEY WERE EVALUATED AFTER 4 WEEKS HEALING.

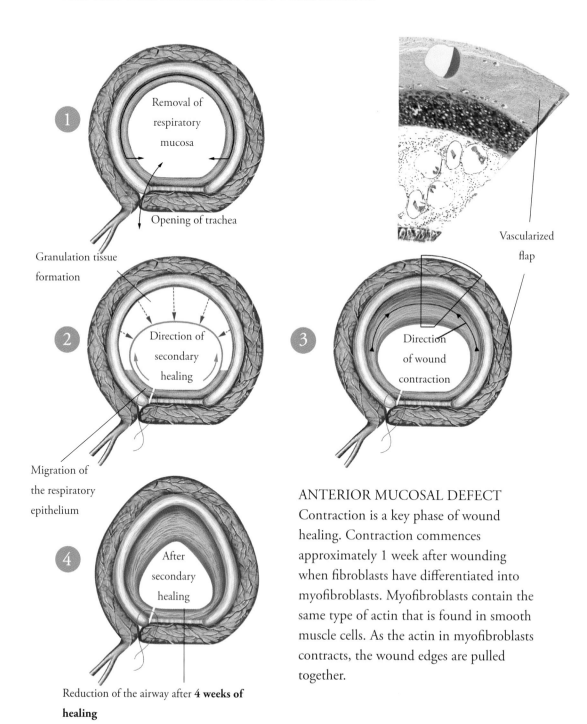

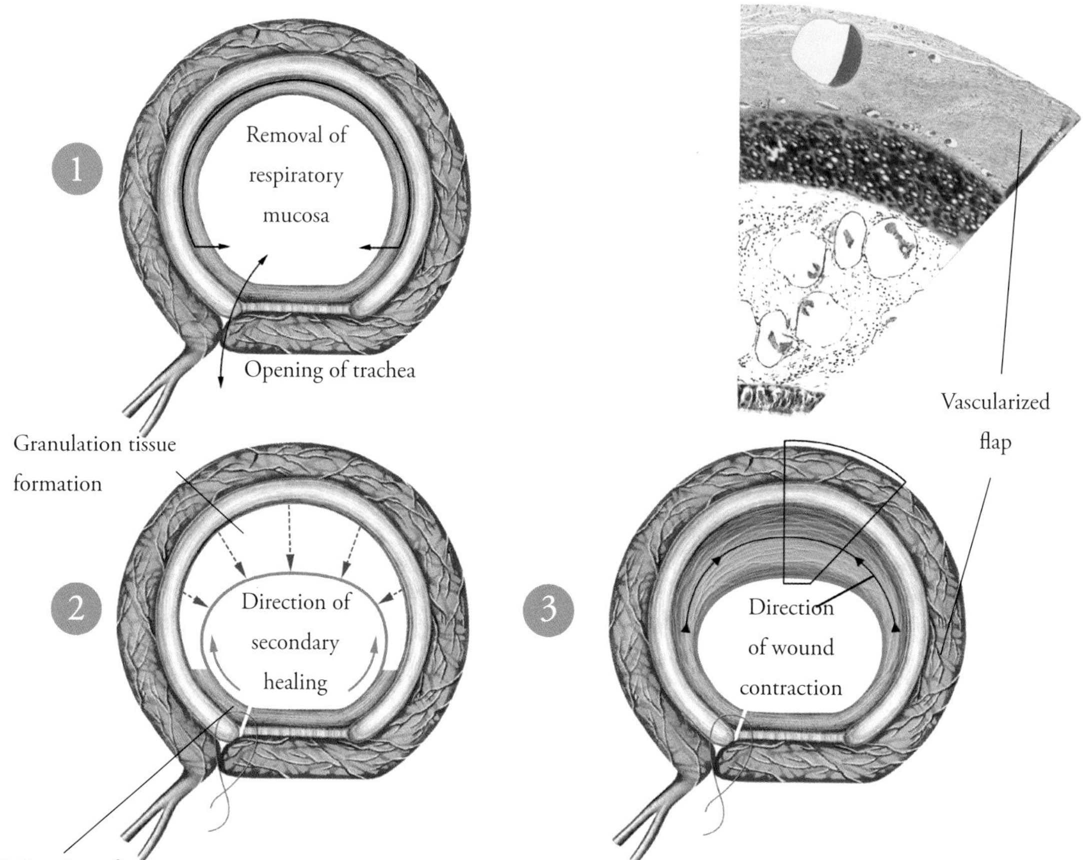
1
Removal of respiratory mucosa
Opening of trachea
Granulation tissue formation
2
Direction of secondary healing
Migration of the respiratory epithelium
3
Direction of wound contraction
Vascularized flap

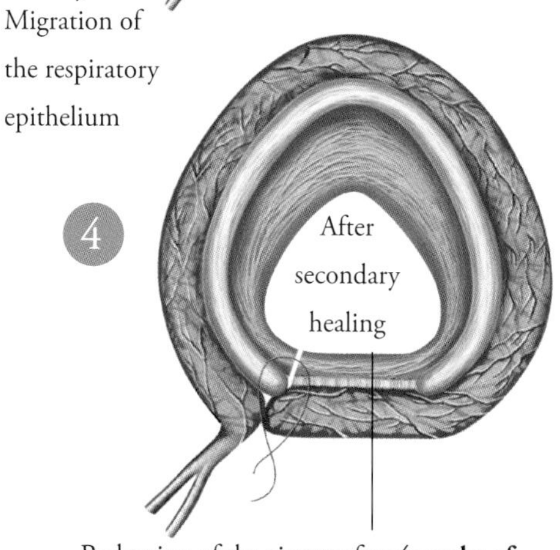
4
After secondary healing

Reduction of the airway after **4 weeks of healing**

ANTERIOR MUCOSAL DEFECT

Contraction is a key phase of wound healing. Contraction commences approximately 1 week after wounding when fibroblasts have differentiated into myofibroblasts. Myofibroblasts contain the same type of actin that is found in smooth muscle cells. As the actin in myofibroblasts contracts, the wound edges are pulled together.

ANIMALS WITH A CIRCUMFERENTIAL DEFECT SHOWED RESPIRATORY DISTRESS AFTER 2 WEEKS OF HEALING AND WERE EVALUATED AT THAT TIME.

FULL-THICKNESS MUCOSAL AIRWAY DEFECT

Healing of these full-thickness wounds combines wound contraction, granulation tissue formation, and reepithelialization from the wound edges. Granulation tissue formation is blocked after being covered by the respiratory epithelial cells. The healing of full-thickness wounds occurs from the periphery of the wound. A fibrin clot is formed and is initially replaced by granulation tissue and later by migrating epithelium from the wound margins. This process is accelerated by wound contraction.
The delay in wound reepithelialization, as a result of limited airway wound contraction of the cartilaginous trachea, results in the production of excessive granulation tissue.

CIRCUMFERENTIAL DEFECT

After **2 weeks of healing**, the longitudinal histology at the anastomosis with the native trachea shows excessive granulation tissue formation over the denuded segment.

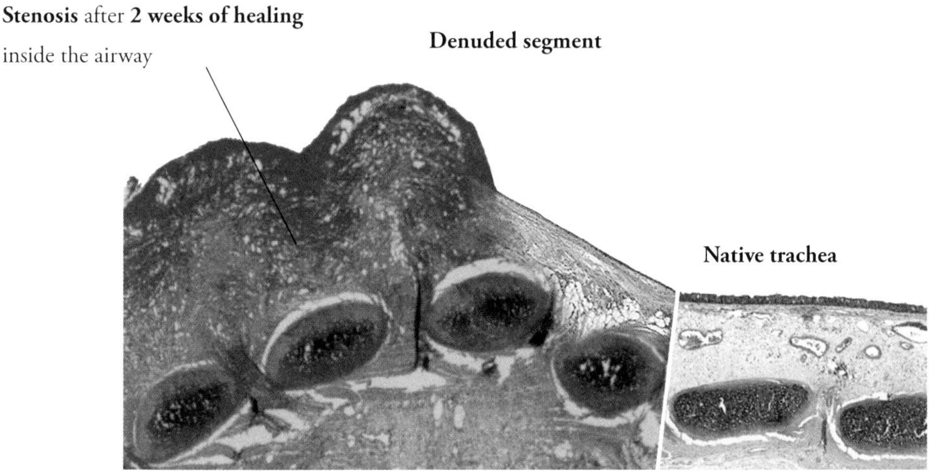
Stenosis after **2 weeks of healing**
inside the airway
Denuded segment
Native trachea

"Secondary healing of a revascularized trachea resulted in the reduction of the airway lumen for partial defects and led to complete stenosis in the circumferential defects."

"The reduction of the airway lumen results of both the excessive granulation tissue formation and wound contraction."

"The migration of respiratory cells is a relatively slow process in full-thickness mucosal wounds."

Mucosal-lined reconstruction

Anterior mucosal defect

The wound area consists of denuded, vascularized cartilage rings and intercartilaginous ligaments.

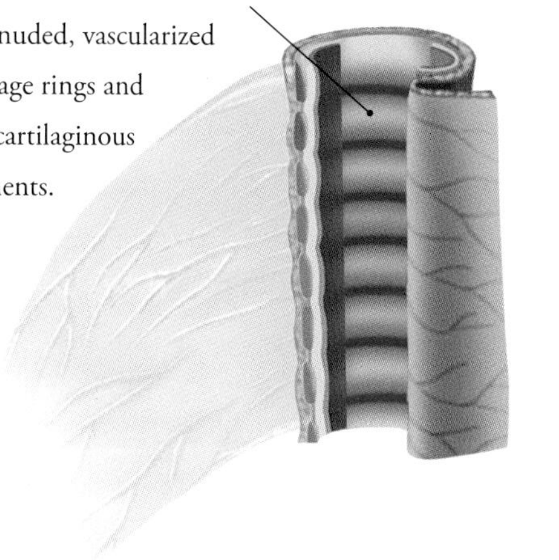

Anterior mucosal graft

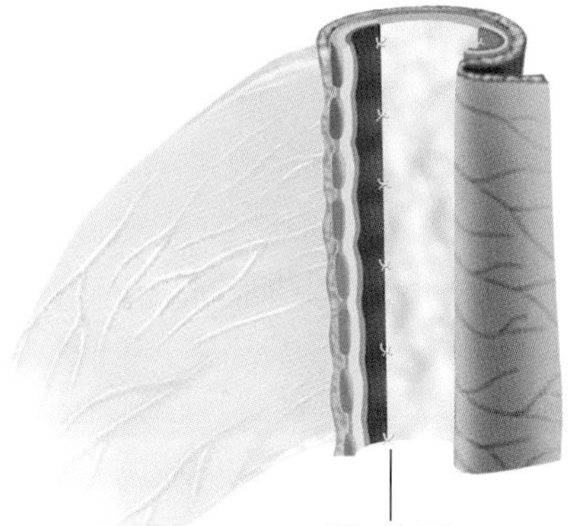
Vicryl 6.0

MUCOSAL GRAFTING

After removal of the respiratory mucosal lining, the denuded patch is grafted with full-thickness buccal mucosa. After mucosal grafting, the tracheal autotransplant can be re-introduced into the airway tract.

A revascularized internal site (cartilage and intercartilaginous ligaments) is essential for the buccal mucosa graft to take.

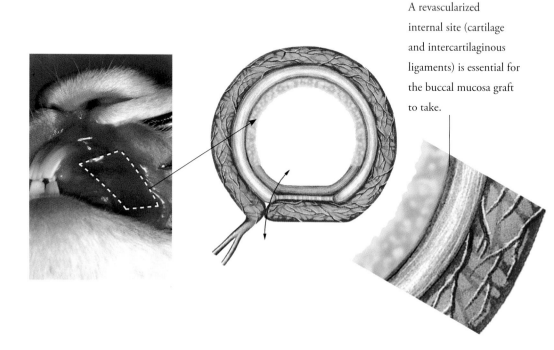

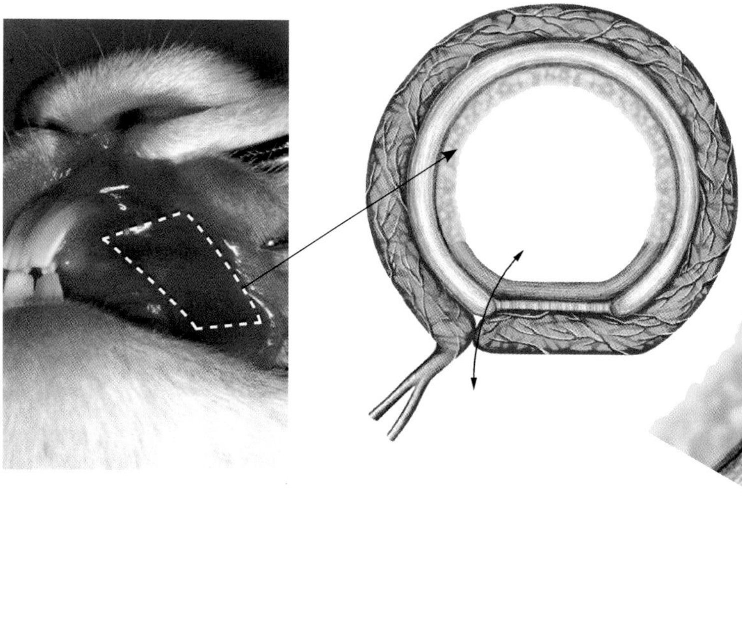

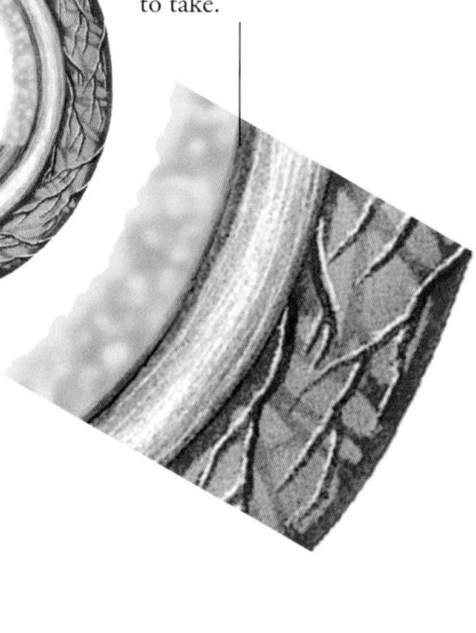

SIMILAR TO THE FULL-THICKNESS SKIN GRAFT, THE MOST EFFECTIVE WAY TO PREVENT THE ADVERSE EFFECTS OF SECONDARY HEALING IS TO COVER THE DEFECT WITH A FULL-THICKNESS MUCOSAL GRAFT. FULL-THICKNESS BUCCAL MUCOSA GRAFTS CAN BE PLACED INSIDE AN ANTERIOR TRACHEAL DEFECT THAT WAS CREATED AFTER ORTHOTOPICAL REVASCULARIZATION. FULL-THICKNESS MUCOSAL GRAFTS INHIBIT WOUND CONTRACTION, THEREBY ALLOWING THE HEALING PROCESS TO PROCEED TOWARDS A MORE REGENERATIVE/LESS SCARRING PATHWAY.

HISTOLOGY OF A DEFECT COVERED WITH A MUCOSAL GRAFT (4 WEEKS AFTER RE-INTRODUCTION INTO THE AIRWAY TRACT)

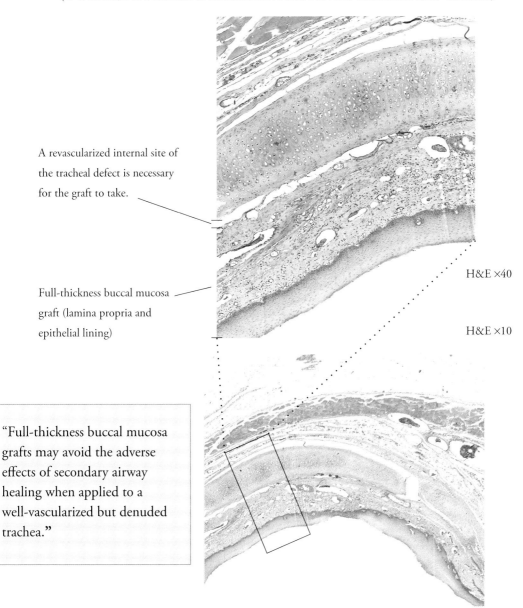

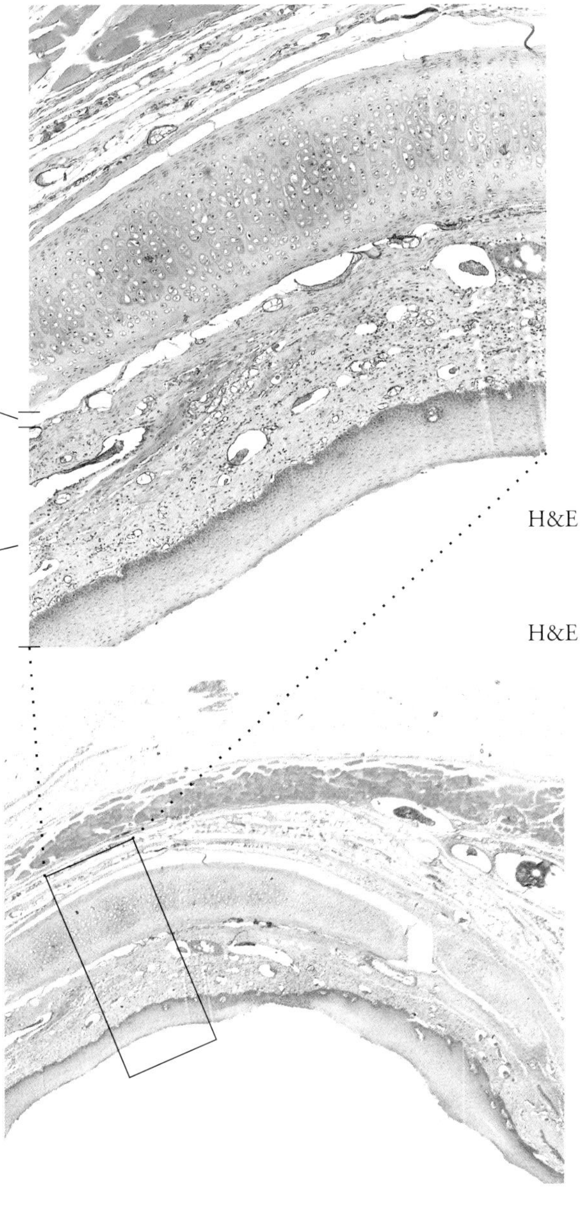
A revascularized internal site of the tracheal defect is necessary for the graft to take.
Full-thickness buccal mucosa graft (lamina propria and epithelial lining)
H&E ×40
H&E ×10

> "Full-thickness buccal mucosa grafts may avoid the adverse effects of secondary airway healing when applied to a well-vascularized but denuded trachea."

Computer technology is Ervinck's preferred medium: with a single gesture, he is able to combine the methodical accuracy of a software expert with the freedom that his mind needs as a source of artistic sustenance. The flying capillary networks may suggest composite tissue transplantation.

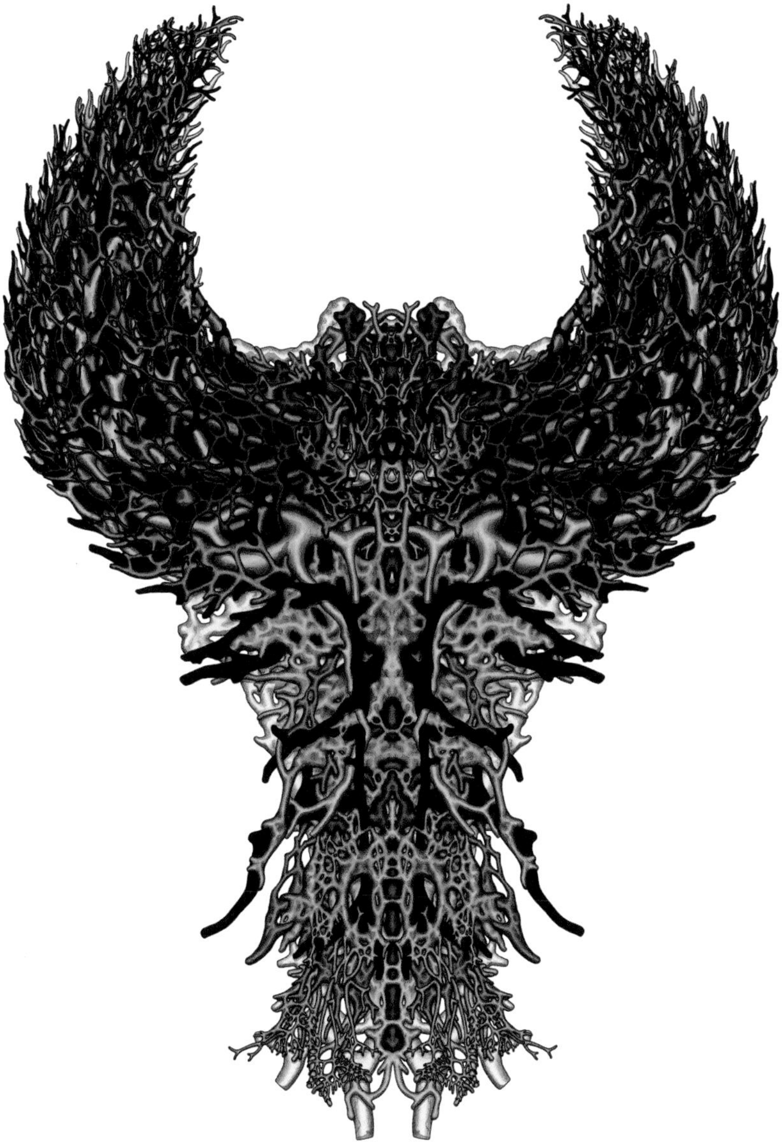

GNITRAORZ, 2010-2011

PRINT

155 × 120 CM

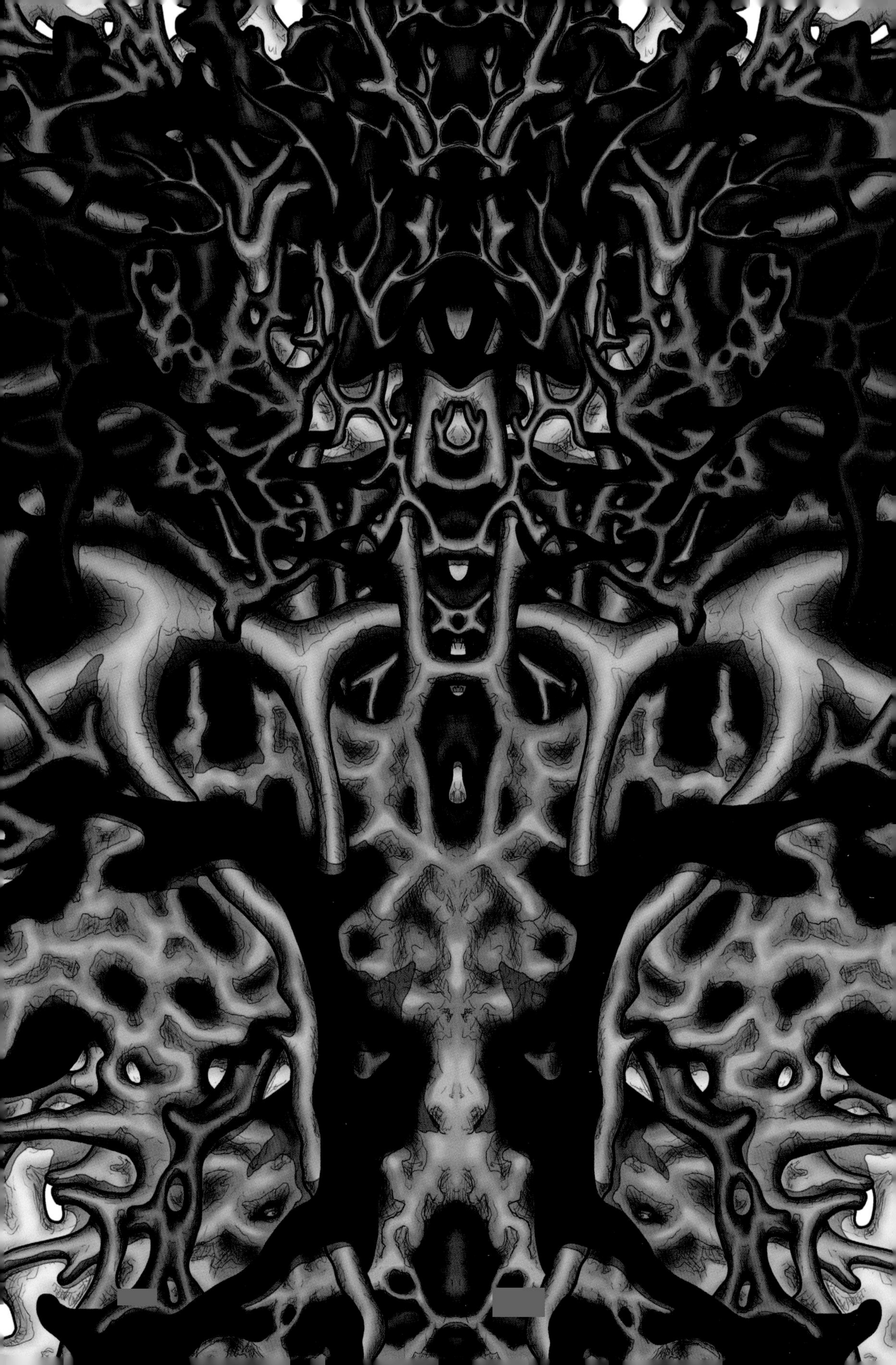

4. Tracheal autotransplantation and laryngeal allotransplantation

---

4.1 Tracheal autotransplantation

Overview

Tumor resection

Tumor resection-CT scan

First stage reconstruction

First stage reconstruction-CT scan

Second stage reconstruction

After tracheal autotransplantation

Second stage reconstruction-CT scan

Closure of the tracheostomy

4.2 Laryngeal allotransplantation

Current knowledge (1) - (2)

Allotransplantation restricted to the larynx (1) - (2)

Tracheal autotransplantation may be used to prevent a total laryngectomy when dealing with an extended hemilaryngectomy defect. The different steps in tracheal autotransplantation are based on a learning curve of more than 75 patients. The first case was performed in 1998.
Laryngeal allotransplantation may be considered to prevent the mutilation of a total laryngectomy defect.

Overview

TRANSPLANTATION OF TRACHEAL SEGMENTS INTO EXTENDED HEMILARYNGECTOMY DEFECTS OCCURS DURING TWO OPERATIONS. TUMOR RESECTION AND ORTHOTOPIC REVASCULARIZATION OCCURS IN A FIRST OPERATION. TRACHEAL AUTOTRANSPLANTATION IS PERFORMED AFTER 2 MONTHS. THE TRACHEOSTOMY CAN USUALLY BE CLOSED AFTER 3 MONTHS.

FIRST OPERATION

The **hyo-epiglottic ligament** is sectioned.

The **anterior commissure** is resected if the tumor reaches the anterior site of the vocal fold.

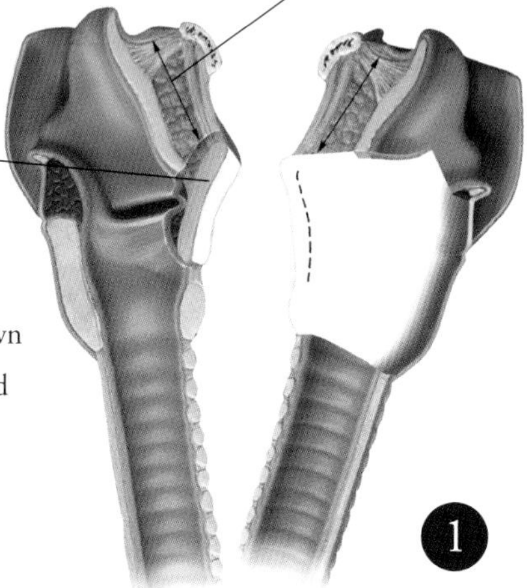
1

The fasciocutaneous paddle is sutured into the laryngeal defect.

The **epiglottis** is pulled down and attached to the thyroid cartilage at the level of the false fold.

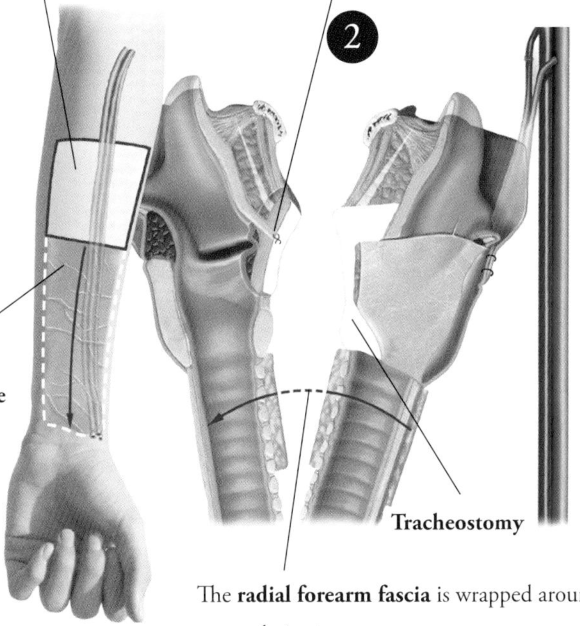
2

The **radial blood vessels** are sutured to the neck vessels.

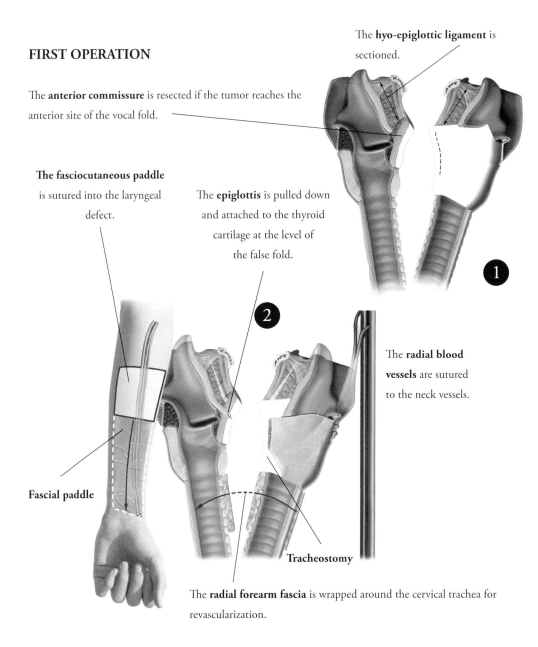

Fascial paddle

Tracheostomy

The **radial forearm fascia** is wrapped around the cervical trachea for revascularization.

SECOND OPERATION

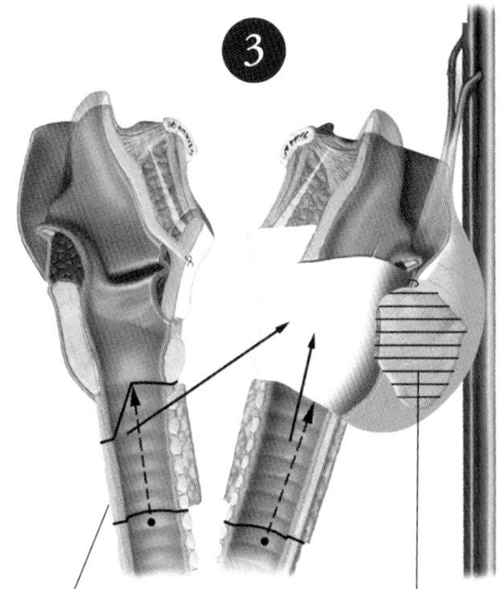
3

The **revascularized trachea** is isolated and transplanted to the laryngeal defect.

The **skin paddle** is removed from the defect and de-epithelialized.

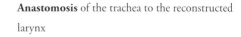

Anastomosis of the trachea to the reconstructed larynx

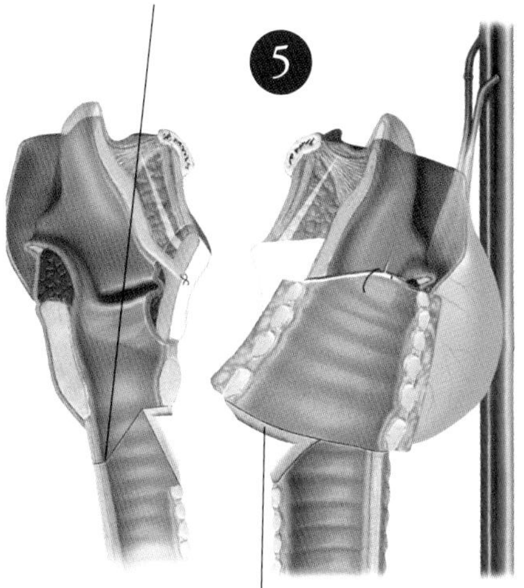
5

The **neck skin flaps** are sutured to the tracheostome.

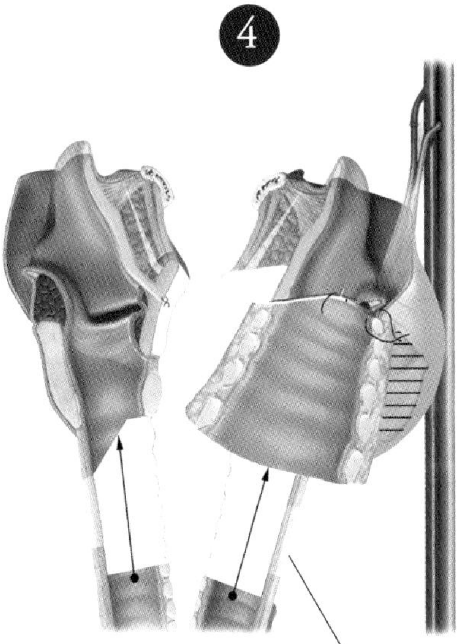
4

A **part of the membranous trachea** is resected to allow for anastomosis (arrows) of the tracheal stump to the reconstructed larynx.

CLOSURE TRACHEOSTOMY

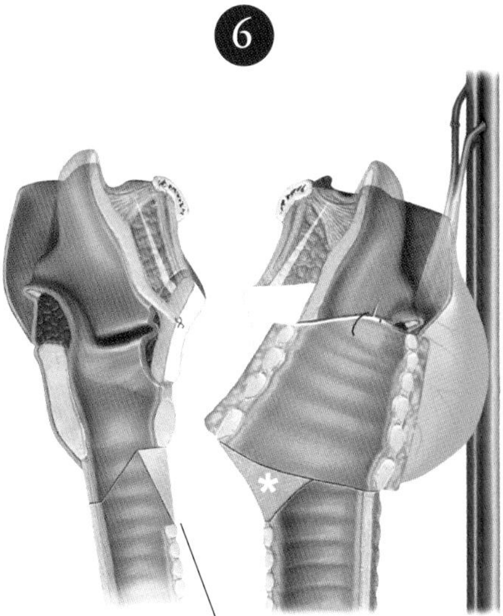
6

Closed tracheostome

The tracheostomy is closed (asterisk) after recovery of all laryngeal functions.

Tumor resection

TUMOR RESECTION FOR A RIGHT T2b-T3 UNILATERAL GLOTTIC CANCER IS SHOWN.

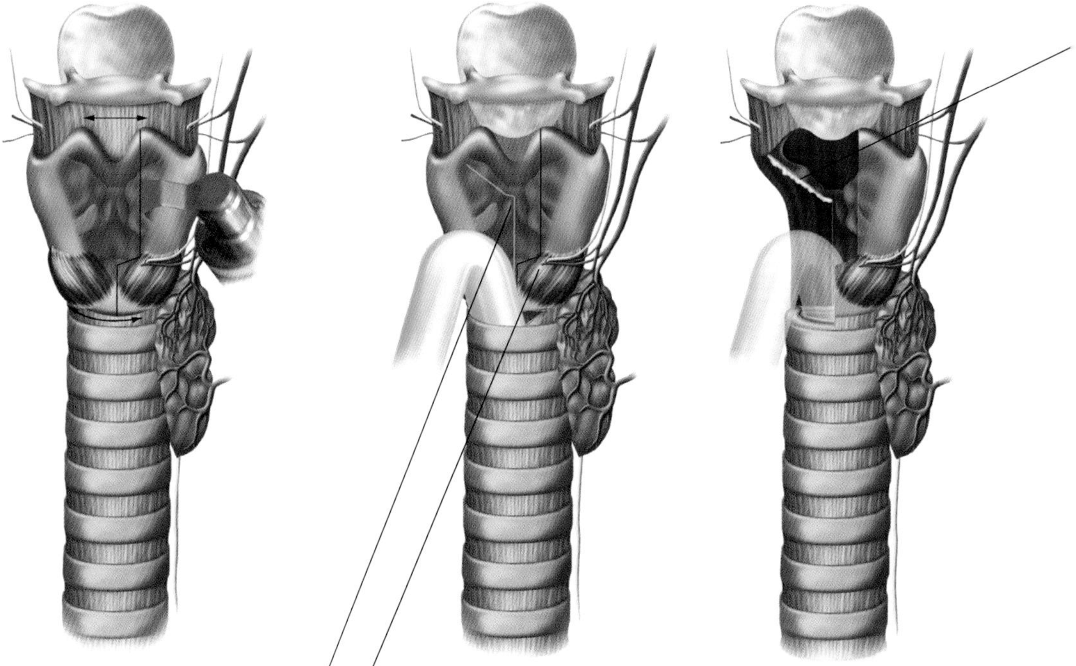

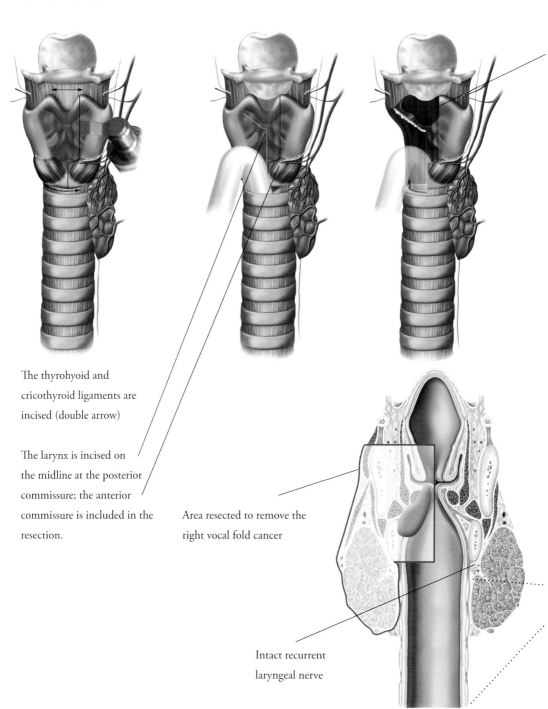

The thyrohyoid and cricothyroid ligaments are incised (double arrow)

The larynx is incised on the midline at the posterior commissure; the anterior commissure is included in the resection.

Area resected to remove the right vocal fold cancer

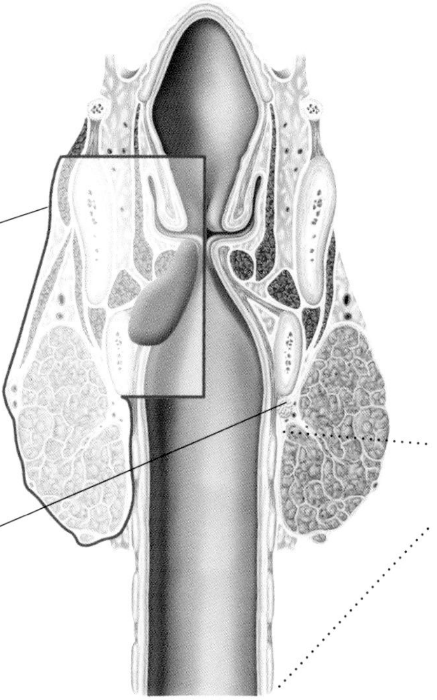

Intact recurrent laryngeal nerve

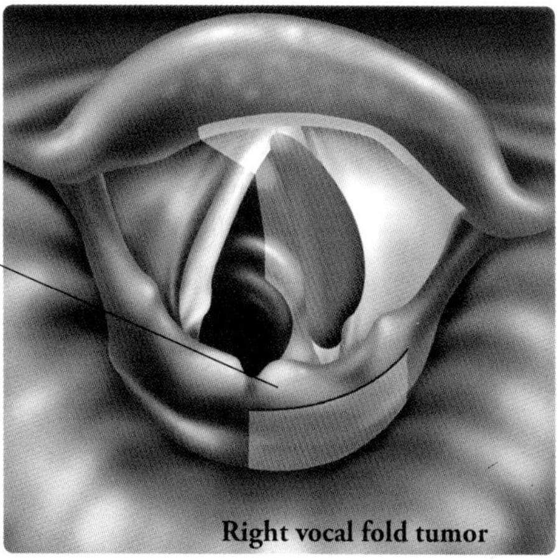
The upper margin of the right aryepiglottic fold is preserved.
Right vocal fold tumor

TRACHEAL SEGMENT USED FOR REVASCULARIZATION

The upper 4 cm of the cervical trachea is dissected from the surrounding thyroid gland to be used for fascial wrapping.

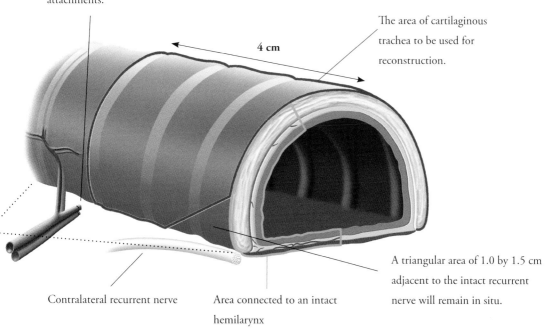

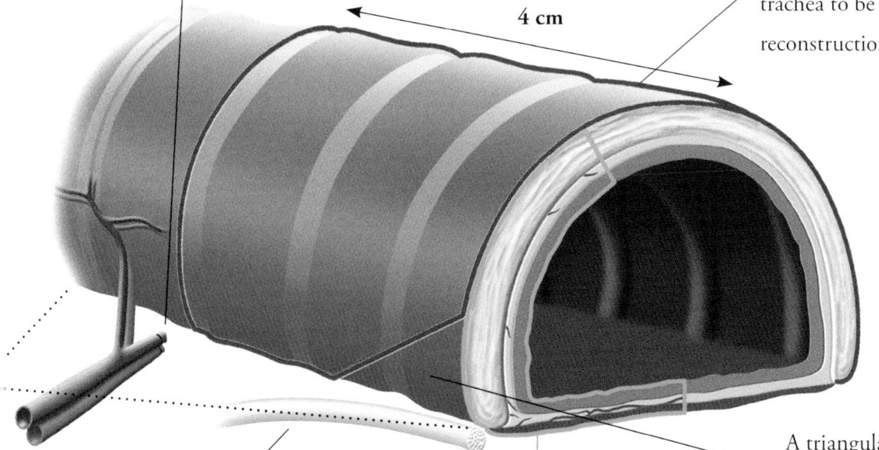
The segmental tracheal blood supply is interrupted after removal of the soft tissue attachments.
4 cm
The area of cartilaginous trachea to be used for reconstruction.
A triangular area of 1.0 by 1.5 cm adjacent to the intact recurrent nerve will remain in situ.
Contralateral recurrent nerve
Area connected to an intact hemilarynx

Tumor resection - CT scan

OVERVIEW ON THE CT SCAN OF AN EXTENDED LARYNGEAL TUMOR AND THE PLANNED RESECTION. THE TUMOR IS A T3 RIGHT VOCAL FOLD CANCER WITH SUBGLOTTIC EXTENSION.

Coronal view

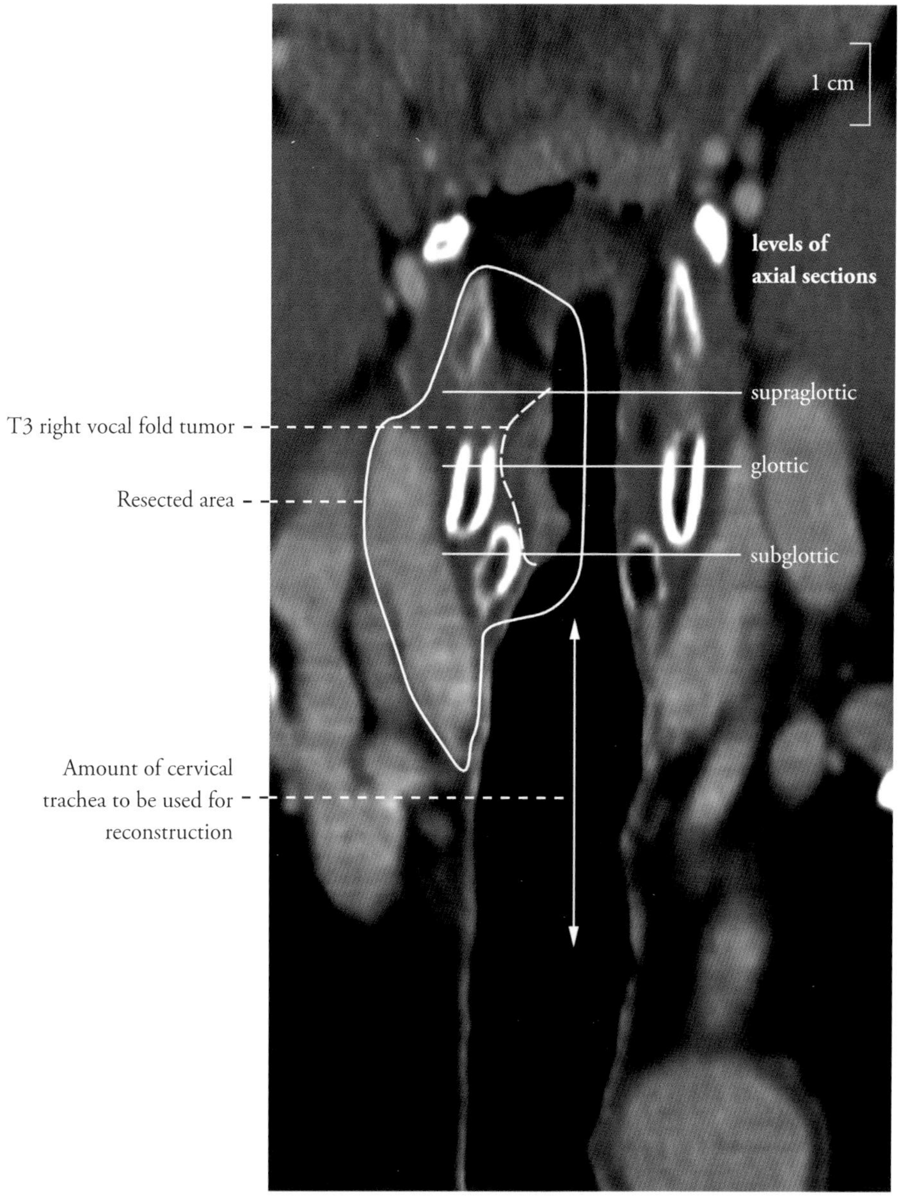
1 cm
levels of axial sections
supraglottic
glottic
subglottic
T3 right vocal fold tumor
Resected area
Amount of cervical trachea to be used for reconstruction

QUIET RESPIRATION PHONATION

Axial view

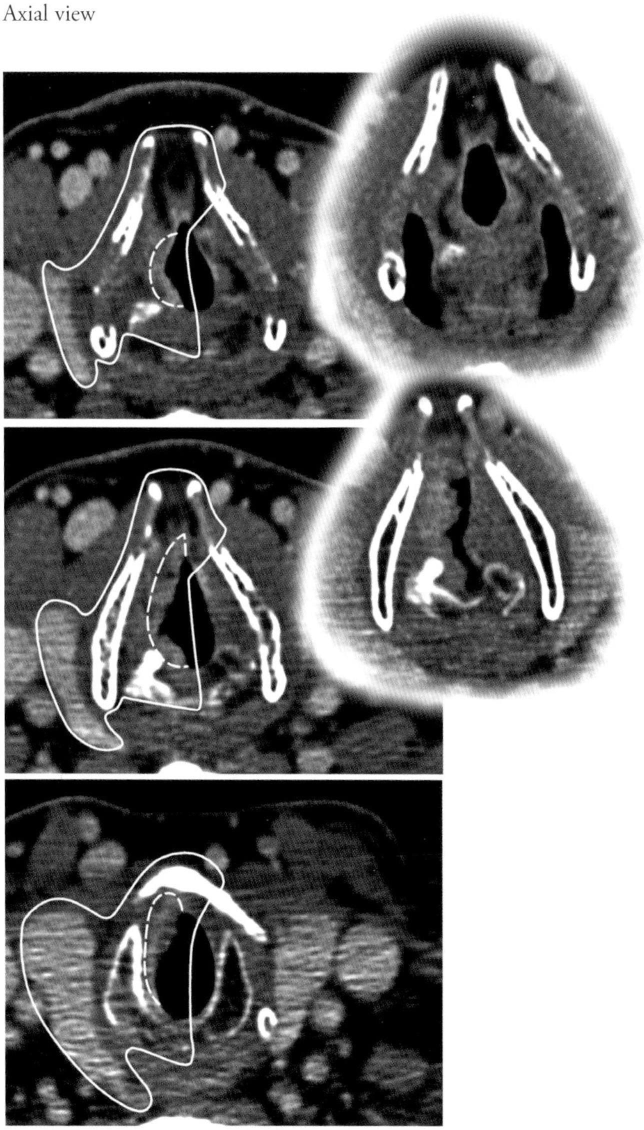

At the **supraglottic level**, the airway lumen size during quiet respiration is identical to the airway lumen size during phonation.

At the **glottic level**, the airway lumen during quiet respiration is more than double the size of the airway lumen during phonation.

On the **CT study during quiet respiration and phonation** (scanning during prolonged phonation of "i"), the laryngeal closure is seen to occur at the glottic level.

First-stage reconstruction

DURING THE FIRST-STAGE OPERATION, THE TUMOR IS RESECTED, THE CERVICAL TRACHEA IS WRAPPED WITH THE RADIAL FOREARM SUBCUTANEOUS TISSUE AND FASCIA AND THE HEMILARYNGEAL DEFECT IS REPAIRED TEMPORARILY WITH THE RADIAL FOREARM SKIN PADDLE. AFTER THIS INTERVENTION, THE PATIENT CAN CLOSE THE GLOTTIC CHINK DURING SPEECH AND SWALLOWING.
A TRACHEOSTOMY IS USED FOR RESPIRATION.

After tumor resection, two sutures (arrows) are placed lateral to the defect, between the epiglottis and the aryepiglottic fold.

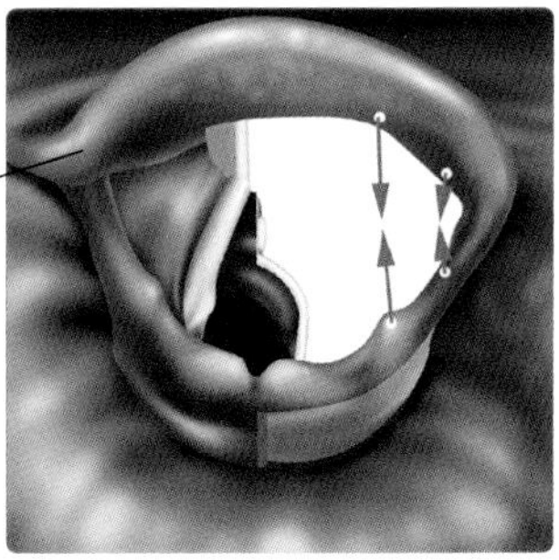

The first lateral side of the skin flap is sutured to the posterior laryngeal section margin, from inferior (black dot) to superior.

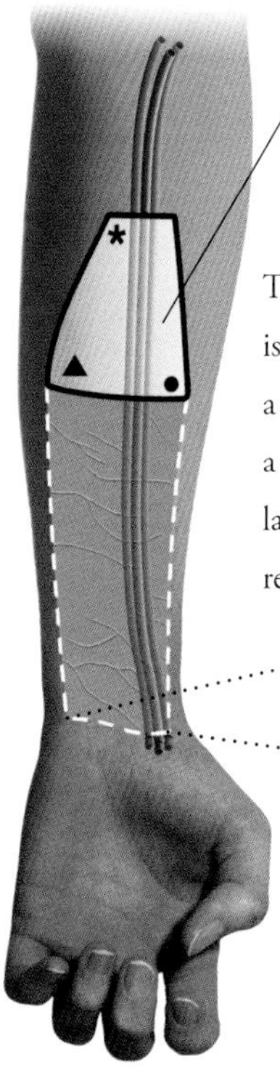

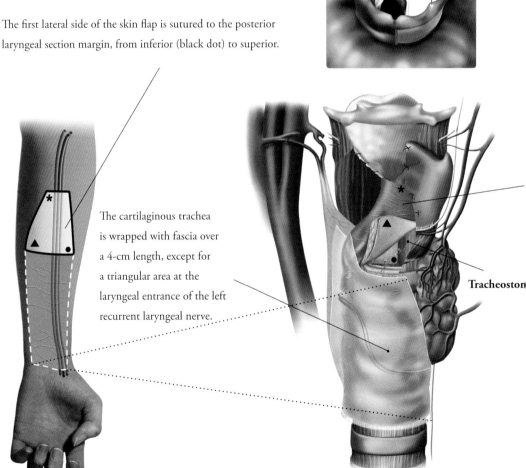

The cartilaginous trachea is wrapped with fascia over a 4-cm length, except for a triangular area at the laryngeal entrance of the left recurrent laryngeal nerve.

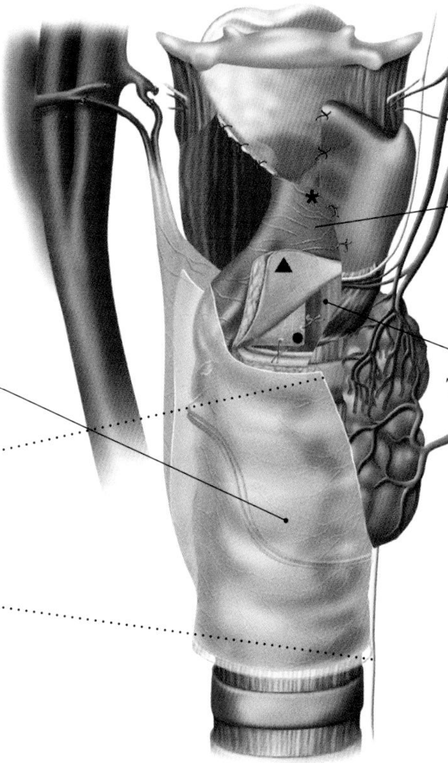
Tracheoston

Sutures are placed to bring the aryepiglottic fold into a position close to the midline.

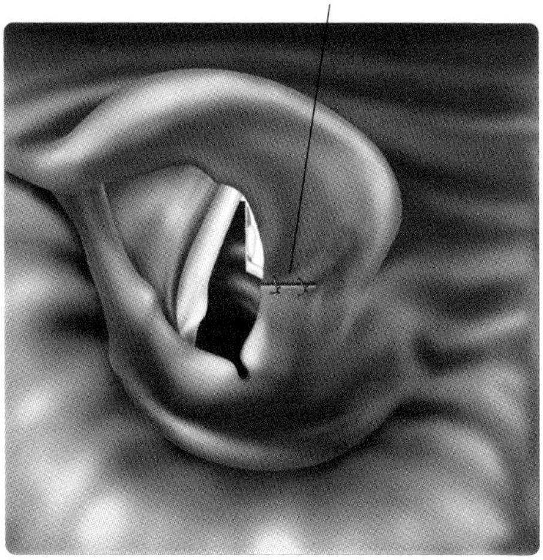

The view after suturing the skin paddle onto the laryngeal defect

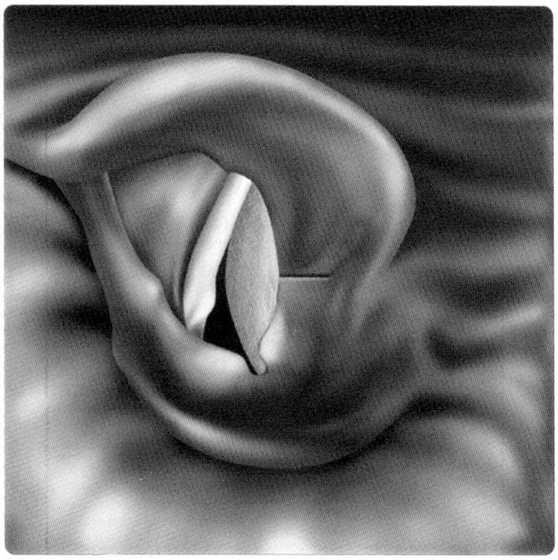

The second lateral side of the skin paddle is sutured to the anterior laryngeal section line, from the superior (asterisk) to the inferior (triangle) aspect. The lower edge (triangle) is not sutured into the laryngeal defect. An opening is left that serves as a tracheostomy.

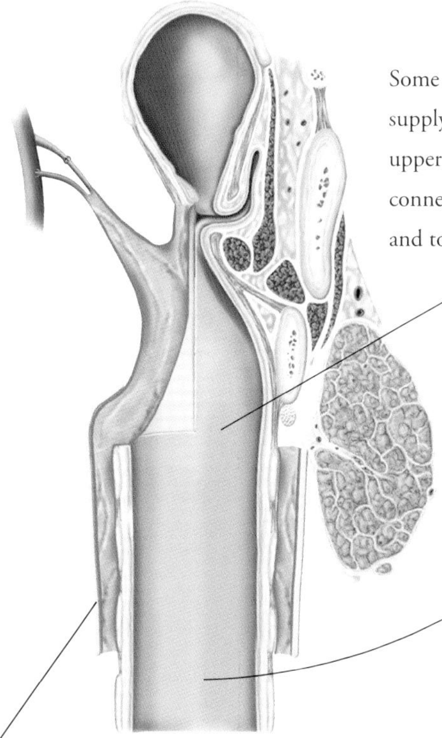

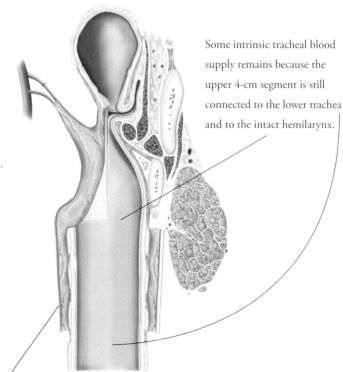

Some intrinsic tracheal blood supply remains because the upper 4-cm segment is still connected to the lower trachea and to the intact hemilarynx.

Gore-tex membrane to prevent adhesions

First stage reconstruction - CT scan

OVERVIEW ON CT SCAN OF TRACHEAL REVASCULARIZATION AND TEMPORARY LARYNX RECONSTRUCTION.

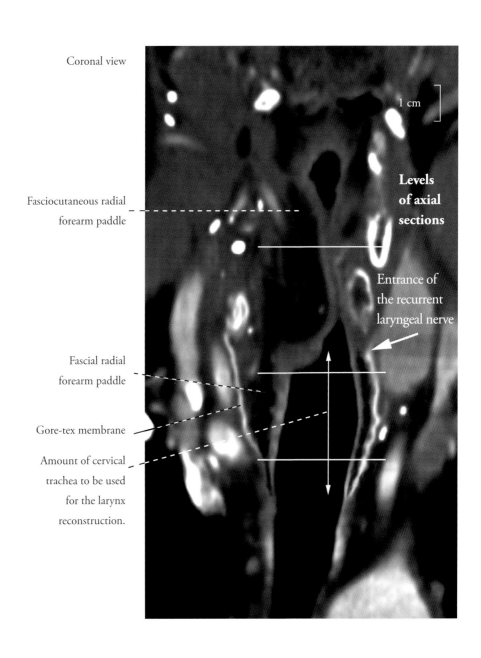

Coronal view

Fasciocutaneous radial forearm paddle

Fascial radial forearm paddle

Gore-tex membrane

Amount of cervical trachea to be used for the larynx reconstruction.

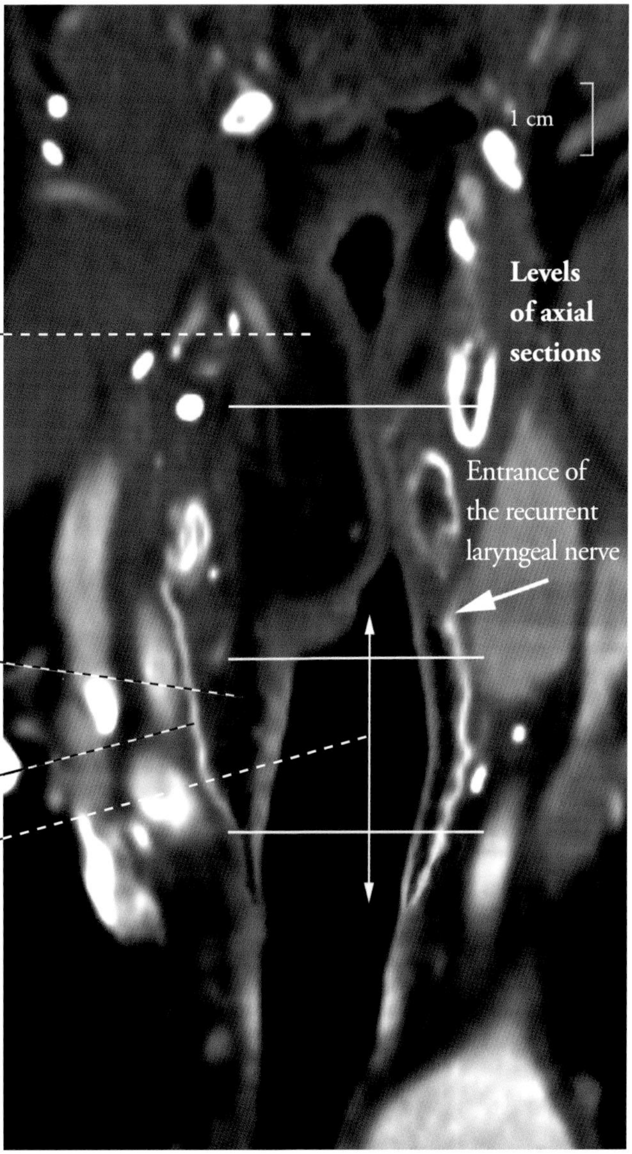
1 cm
Levels of axial sections
Entrance of the recurrent laryngeal nerve

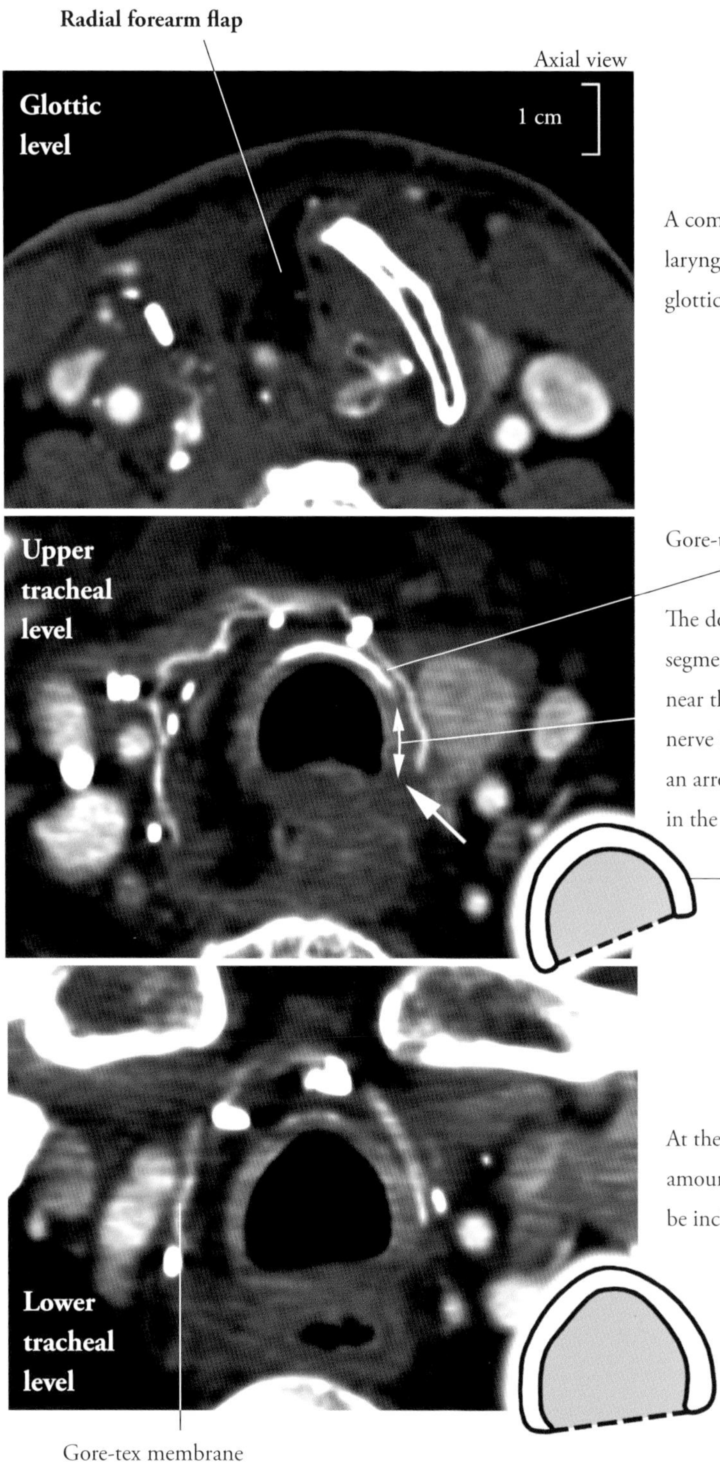
Radial forearm flap
Axial view
Glottic level
1 cm
Upper tracheal level
Lower tracheal level
Gore-tex membrane

A complete obliteration of the laryngeal lumen is visible at the glottic level.

Gore-tex membrane

The double arrow shows a 1-cm segment of the cervical trachea near the recurrent laryngeal nerve (position indicated with an arrow), which is not included in the autotransplant.

This section shows the amount of cartilaginous trachea that will be included in the autotransplant.

At the lower tracheal level, the full amount of cartilaginous trachea will be included in the autotransplant.

Second stage reconstruction

DURING THE SECOND STAGE OPERATION (USUALLY 2 MONTHS AFTER THE FIRST INTERVENTION), THE SKIN PADDLE IS REMOVED FROM THE LARYNGEAL DEFECT AND DE-EPITHELIALIZED. THE CERVICAL TRACHEA IS AUTOTRANSPLANTED WITH AN INTACT BLOOD SUPPLY TO THE HEMILARYNGEAL DEFECT. THE MEDIASTINAL TRACHEA IS MOBILIZED AND SUTURED TO THE RECONSTRUCTED LARYNX. A TRACHEOSTOMY IS MAINTAINED BETWEEN THE RECONSTRUCTED LARYNX AND THE MEDIASTINAL TRACHEA.

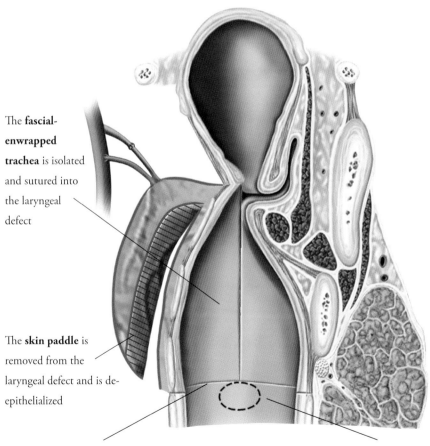

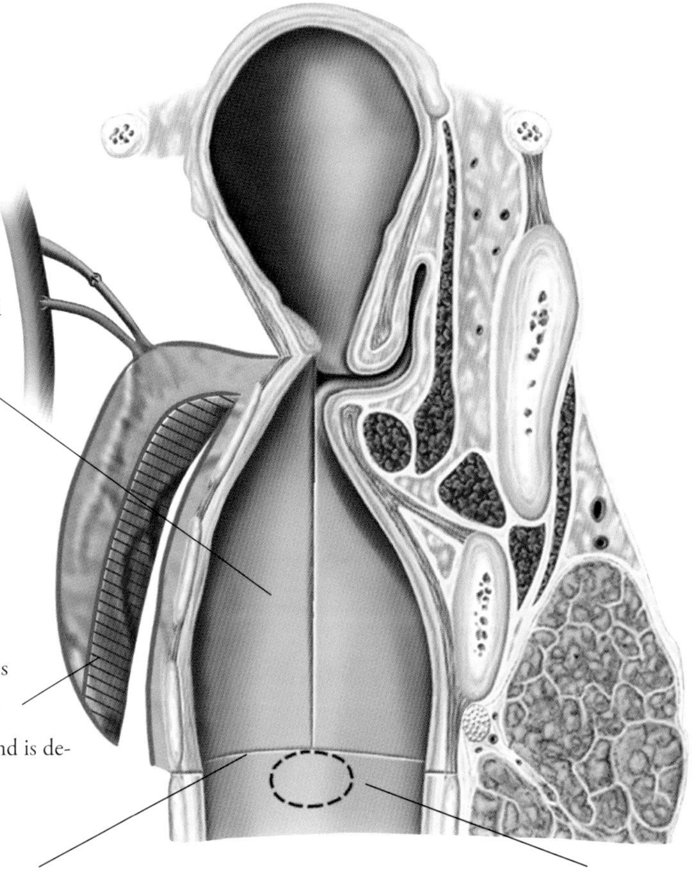
The **fascial-enwrapped trachea** is isolated and sutured into the laryngeal defect
The **skin paddle** is removed from the laryngeal defect and is de-epithelialized
The **airway continuity** is re-established by bringing up the tracheal stump to the lower end of the reconstructed larynx
The tracheostomy is maintained below the reconstructed larynx

ndoscopic laryngeal view after tracheal ıtotransplantation during quiet respiration.

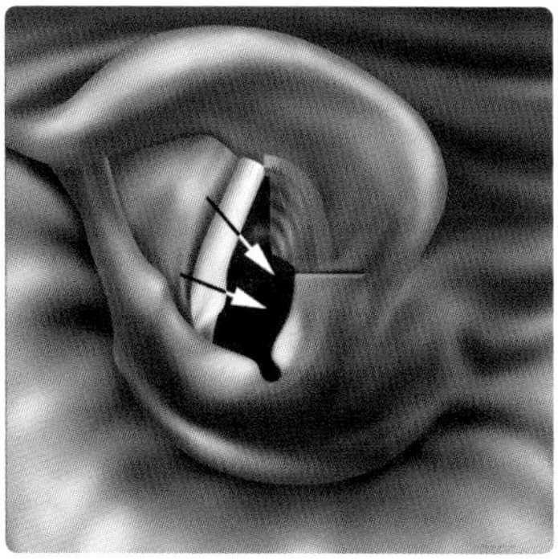

During phonation, closure (arrows) occurs between the false fold and the aryepiglottic fold at the site of resection.

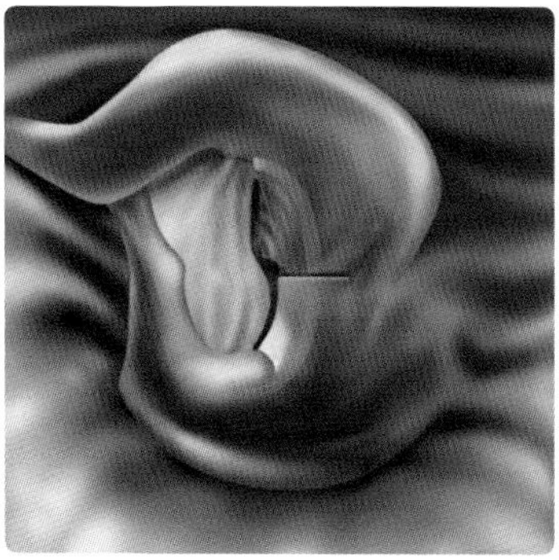

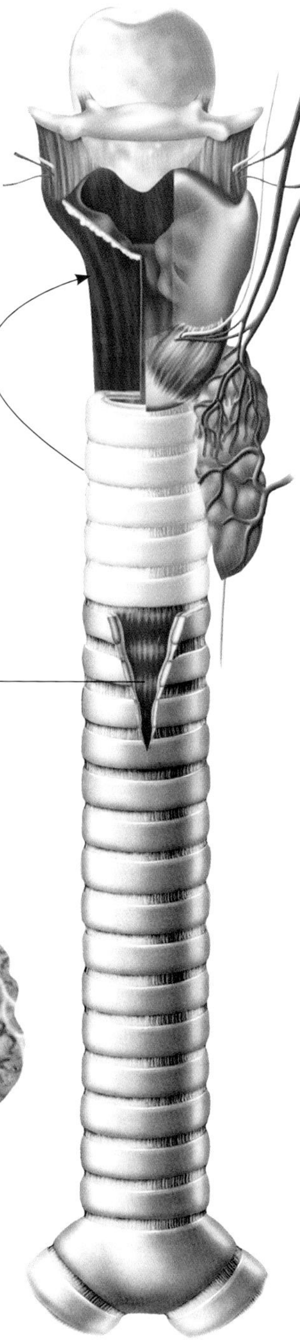
Tracheostomy

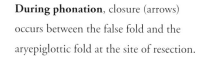

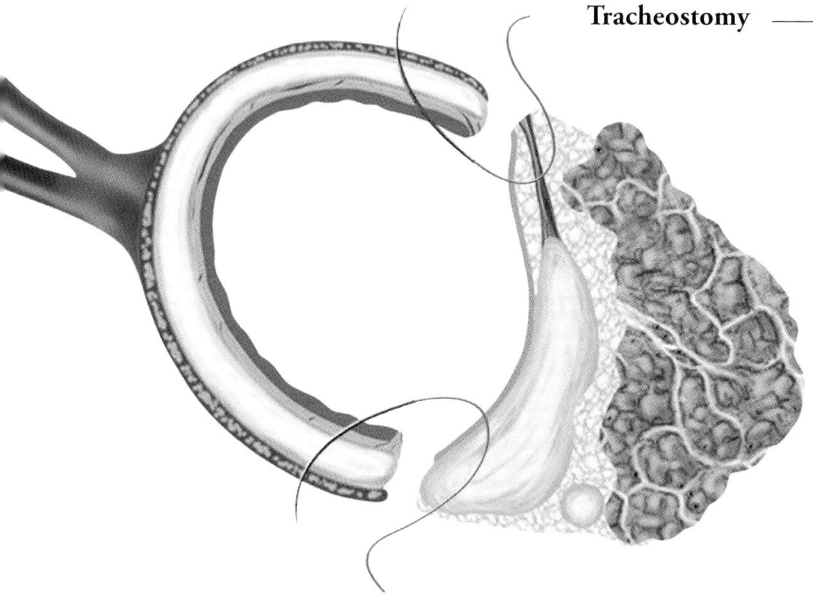
Tracheal autotransplant
Laryngeal remnant

After tracheal autotransplantation

SITUATION AFTER TRACHEAL AUTOTRANSPLANTATION AND AFTER THE ANASTOMOSIS OF THE TRACHEAL STUMP TO THE RECONSTRUCTED LARYNX. A TRACHEOSTOME IS FORMED BY SUTURING THE NECK SKIN FLAPS TO THE ANTERIOR AIRWAY DEFECT.

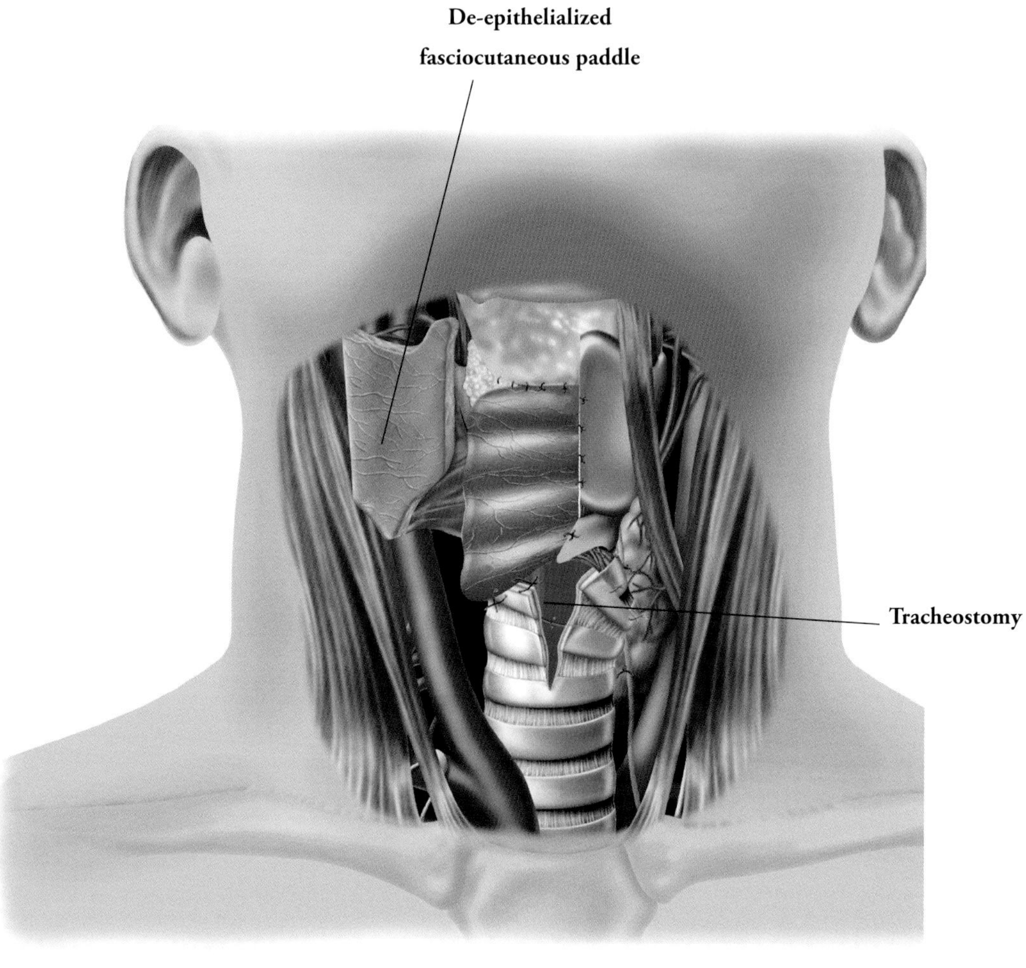
De-epithelialized
fasciocutaneous paddle
Tracheostomy

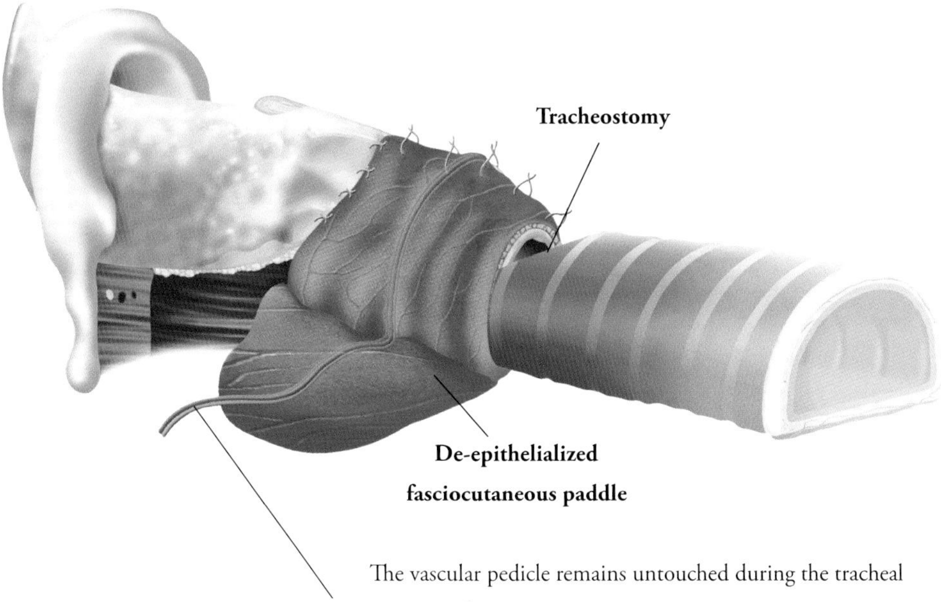
Tracheostomy
De-epithelialized
fasciocutaneous paddle

The vascular pedicle remains untouched during the tracheal autotransplantation.

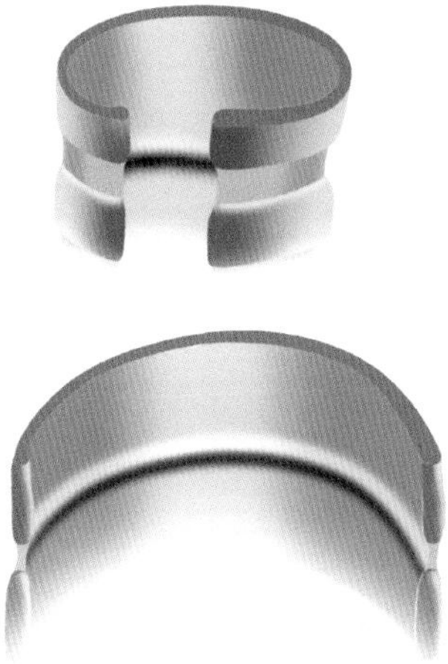

The tracheal cartilage rings are giving support for airway reconstruction. This elastic structure will provide more or less convexity depending on the width of the defect.

Second stage reconstruction - CT scan

OVERVIEW ON CT SCAN AFTER TRACHEAL AUTOTRANSPLANTATION. PHONATION OCCURS AT THE SUPRAGLOTTIC LEVEL, AS CAN BE SEEN ON THE CT SCAN DURING PHONATION.

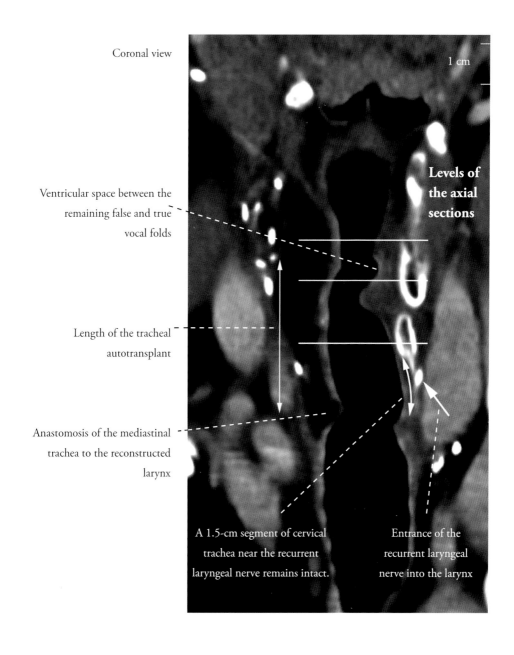

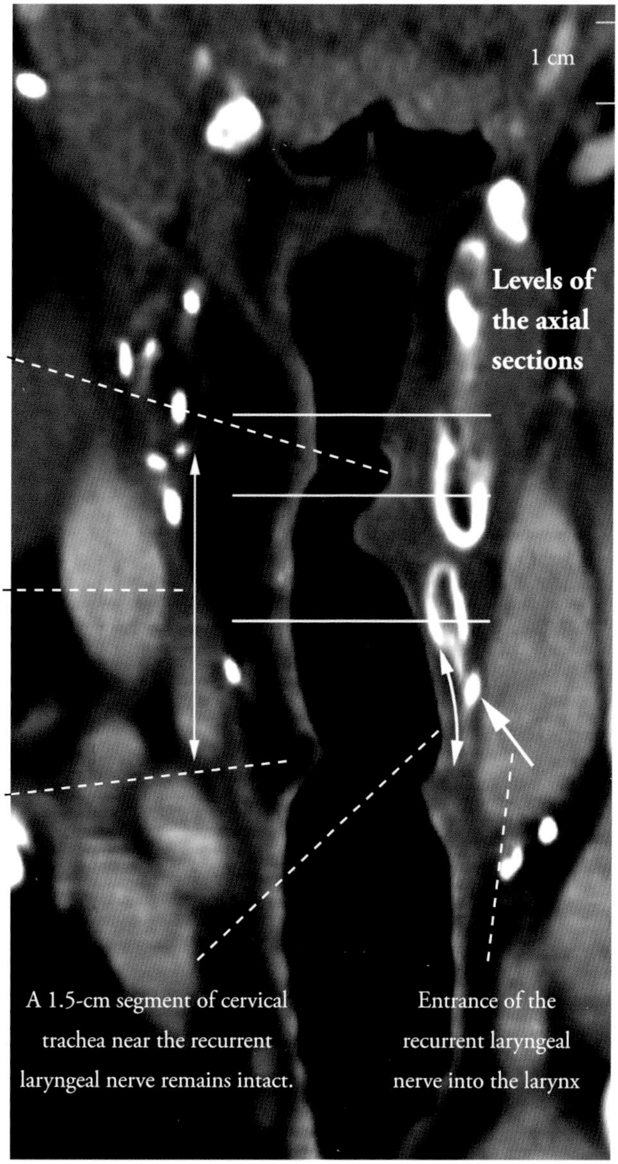
Coronal view
1 cm
Levels of the axial sections
Ventricular space between the remaining false and true vocal folds
Length of the tracheal autotransplant
Anastomosis of the mediastinal trachea to the reconstructed larynx
A 1.5-cm segment of cervical trachea near the recurrent laryngeal nerve remains intact.
Entrance of the recurrent laryngeal nerve into the larynx

At the supraglottic level, the airway lumen during **quiet respiration** is almost eight times larger than the airway lumen during phonation.

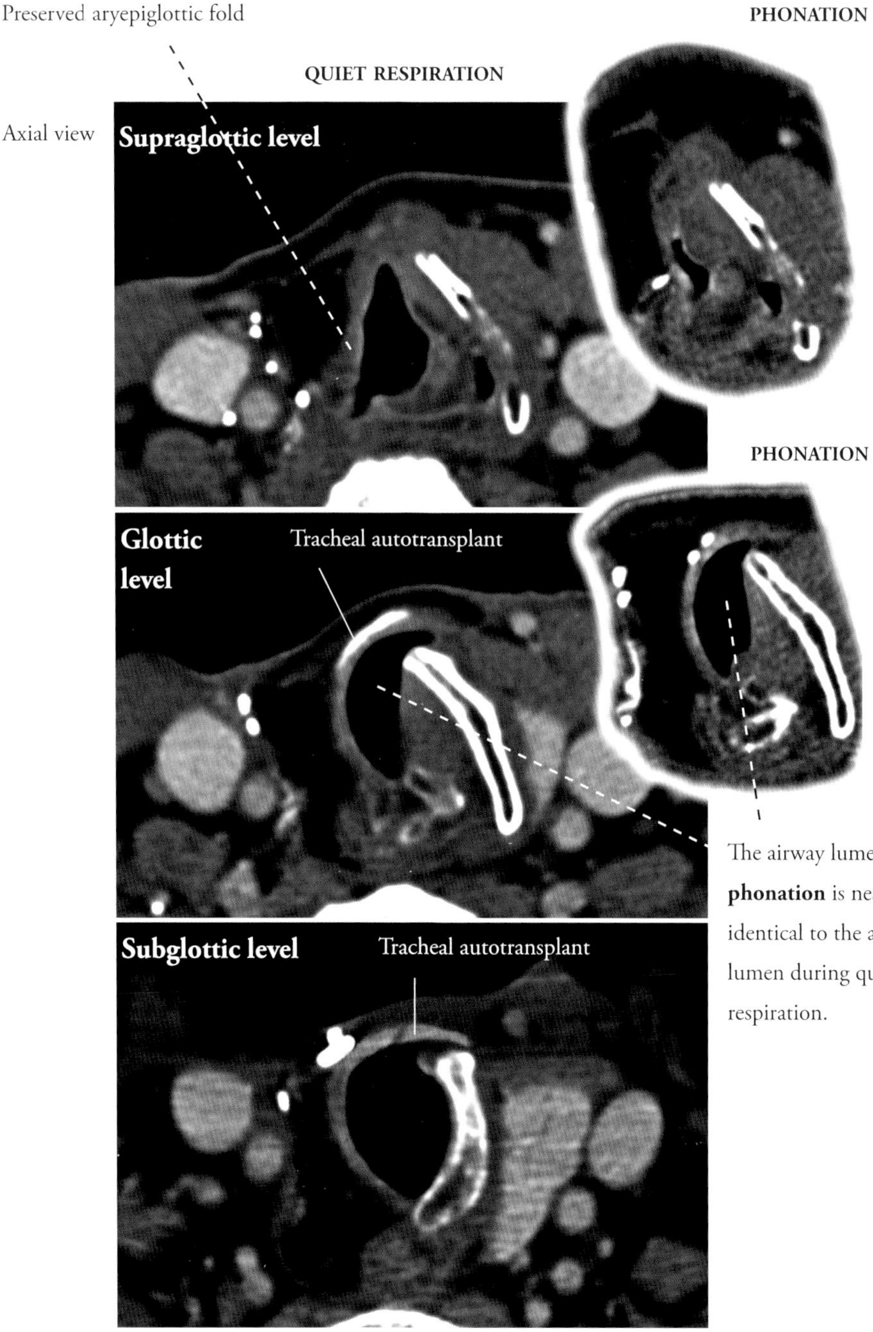
Preserved aryepiglottic fold
PHONATION
QUIET RESPIRATION
Axial view
Supraglottic level
PHONATION
Glottic level
Tracheal autotransplant
Subglottic level
Tracheal autotransplant

The airway lumen during **phonation** is nearly identical to the airway lumen during quiet respiration.

Closure of the tracheostomy

THE TRACHEOSTOMY CAN BE CLOSED AFTER THE FULL RECOVERY OF ALL LARYNGEAL FUNCTIONS, WHICH USUALLY OCCURS FROM 4 TO 8 WEEKS AFTER TRACHEAL AUTOTRANSPLANTATION.

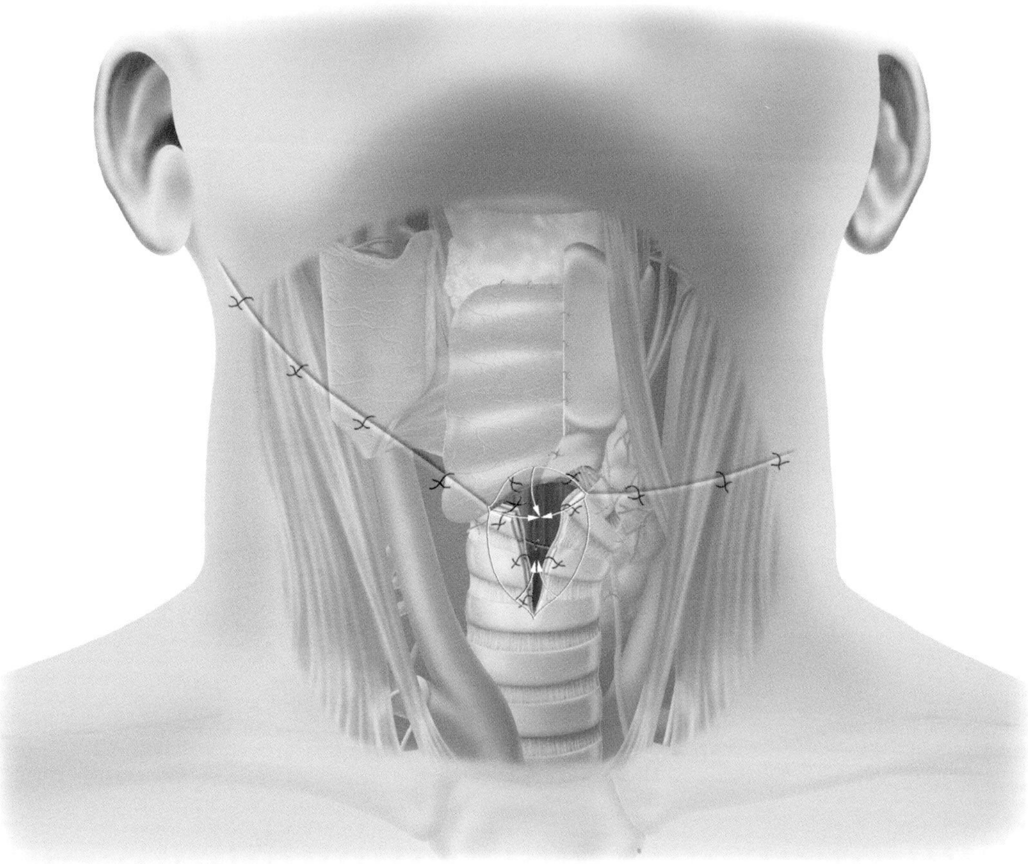

The neck skin around the tracheostomy is incised and inverted (arrows).

TRACHEOSTOMY CLOSURE

After the inversion of the skin flaps. The dotted lines show the circumference of the tracheostome before closure. Arrows show the second layer closure with an upper and lower neck skin flap.

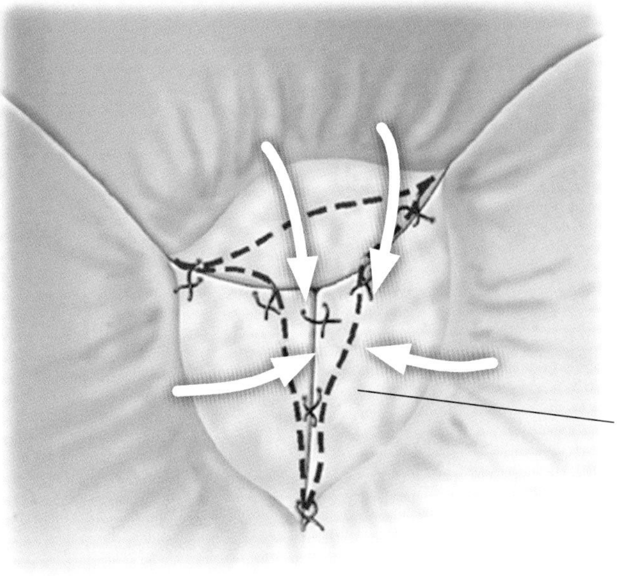

Subcutaneous tissue of the inverted skin flaps

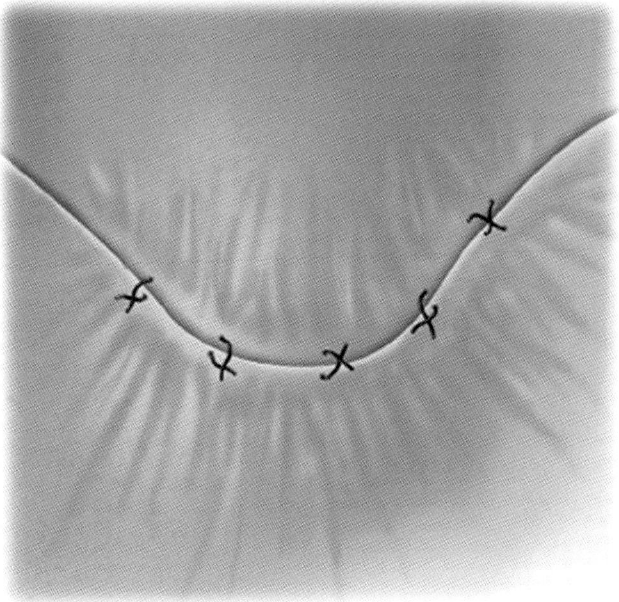

The upper and lower neck skin flaps are undermined and closed as a second layer closure.

> "Tracheal autotransplantation can prevent a total laryngectomy in selected lateralized tumor cases."

Current knowledge (1)

IN LARYNGEAL TRANSPLANTATION, THE MAJOR OBSTACLES TO OVERCOME ARE REVASCULARIZATION, REINNERVATION, AND IMMUNOSUPPRESSION. TO DATE, TWO TRANSPLANTATIONS HAVE BEEN PERFORMED IN THE USA*. LARYNGEAL STENOSIS WAS THE REASON FOR TRANSPLANTATION IN BOTH CASES. THE TWO PATIENTS UNDERWENT TRANSPLANTATION OF THE LARYNX, CERVICAL TRACHEA, PHARYNX, AND THE THYROID AND PARATHYROID GLANDS.

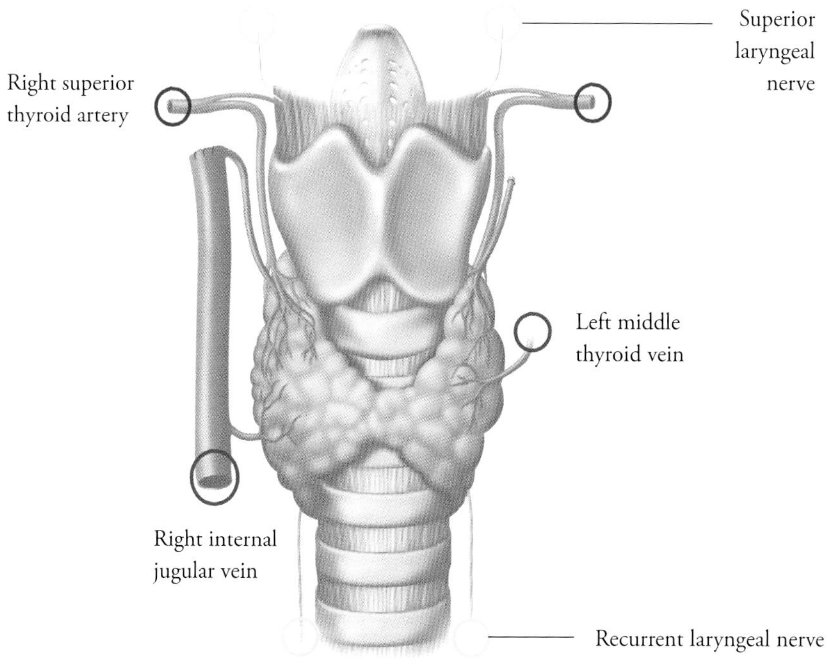
Superior laryngeal nerve
Right superior thyroid artery
Left middle thyroid vein
Right internal jugular vein
Recurrent laryngeal nerve

Laryngeal allotransplant

LARYNGEAL ALLOTRANSPLANTATION

The donor's right superior thyroid artery can be anastomosed to that of the recipient (end-to-end anastomosis), and the proximal end of the donor's right internal jugular vein can be anastomosed to the recipient's right internal jugular vein (end-to-side). The left anastomoses include the donor's superior thyroid artery to the recipient's superior thyroid artery (end-to-end) and the donor's middle thyroid vein to the recipient's internal jugular vein (end-to-side). Both the superior laryngeal nerves and recurrent laryngeal nerves should be anastomosed.

THE TOTAL LARYNGECTOMY DEFECT

The rationale for transplanting not only the larynx but also the cervical trachea, thyroid, and parathyroid glands can be found in the total laryngectomy defect performed on patients with locally advanced or recurrent squamous cell carcinoma. This defect includes a 2 cm segment of the cervical trachea. However, at present, because of the increased risk of a second cancer, patients who have been treated for laryngeal cancer should not be considered suitable for larynx transplantation.

Total laryngectomy defect

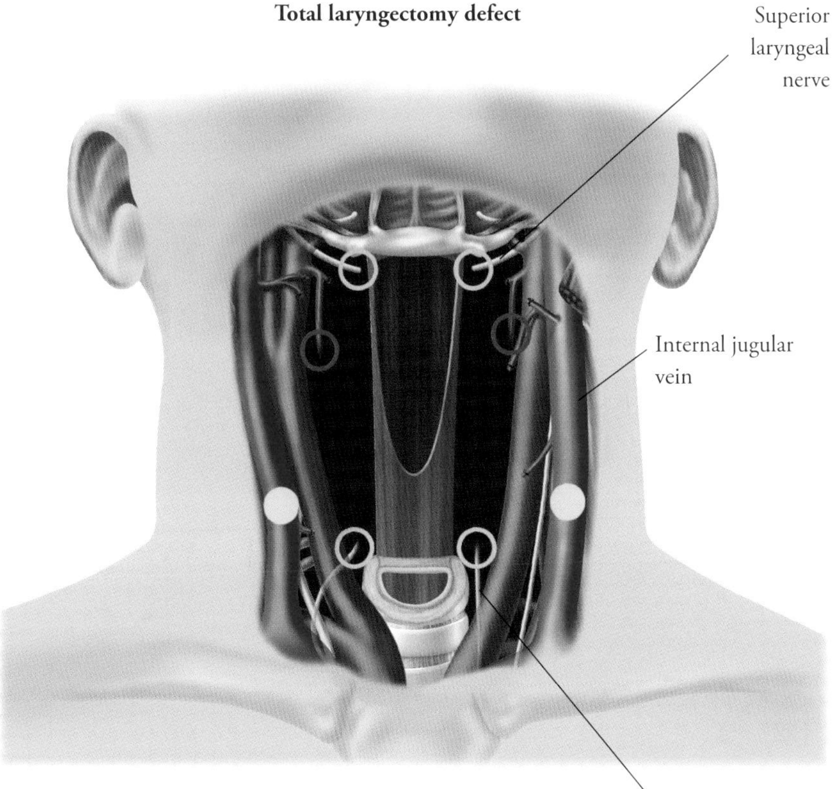
Superior laryngeal nerve
Internal jugular vein
Recurrent laryngeal nerve

* 1. Strome M. et al. New Engl J Med 2001;344:1676-1679.
2. http://www.ucdmc.ucdavis.edu/otolaryngology/

Current knowledge (2)

THE FULL REVASCULARIZATION OF THE ALLOGRAFT WAS OBTAINED AND MAINTAINED WITH THE DAILY ADMINISTRATION OF IMMUNOSUPPRESSION. THREE MONTHS POST-TRANSPLANTATION, THE SUPRAGLOTTIS AND VOCAL FOLDS WERE SENSITIVE TO TOUCH, AND THE SWALLOWING FUNCTION HAD RETURNED. THEY WERE UNABLE TO BREATHE WITHOUT A CANNULA DUE TO THE MIDLINE POSITION OF THE VOCAL FOLDS. BOTH PATIENTS BELIEVE THAT THEIR QUALITY OF LIFE IMPROVED NOTABLY.

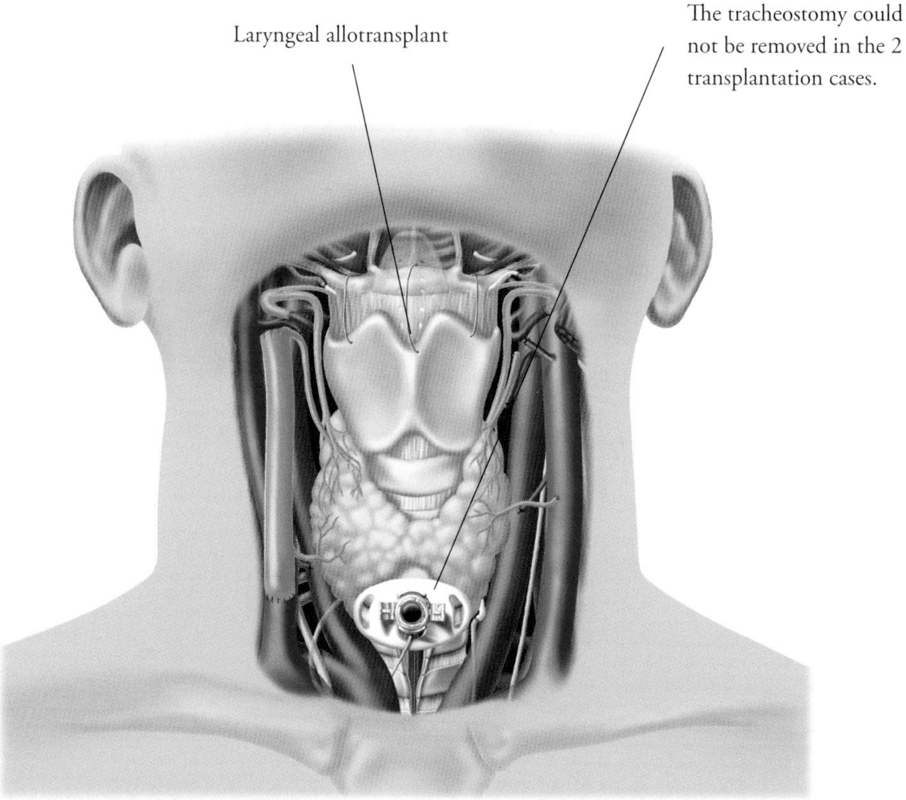
Laryngeal allotransplant
The tracheostomy could not be removed in the 2 transplantation cases.

"Problematic motor reinnervation with the impossibility of opening the glottic chink during respiration and the necessity for continuous immunosuppression are the main reasons why it is doubtful that larynx allotransplantation in the presented form will play a role in the reconstruction of total laryngeal defects in the near future."

MORPHOLOGY AFTER LARYNGEAL ALLOTRANSPLANTATION

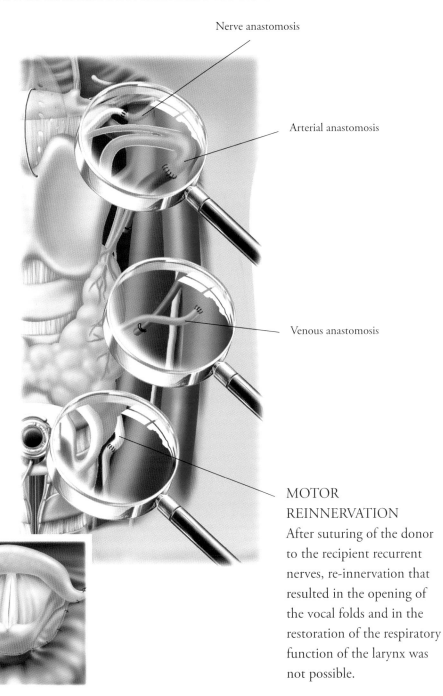

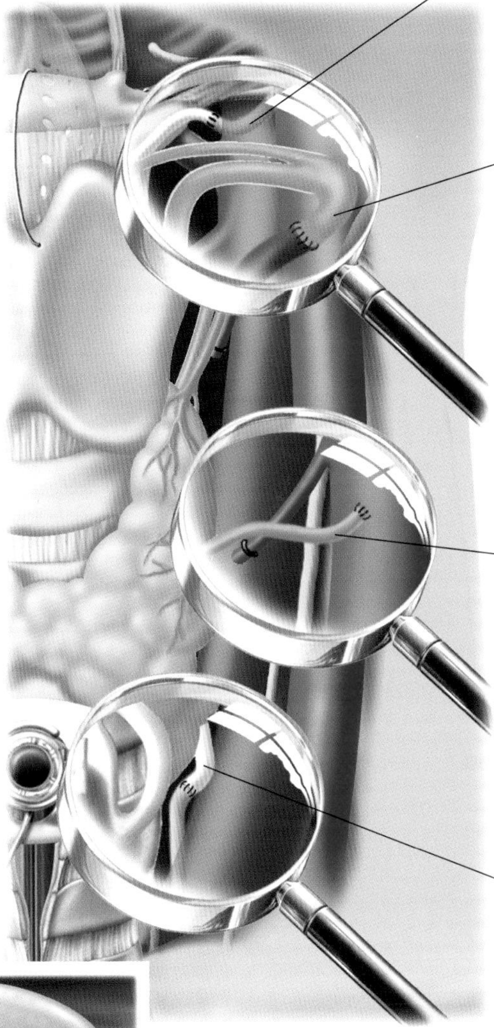
Nerve anastomosis
Arterial anastomosis
Venous anastomosis

MOTOR REINNERVATION
After suturing of the donor to the recipient recurrent nerves, re-innervation that resulted in the opening of the vocal folds and in the restoration of the respiratory function of the larynx was not possible.

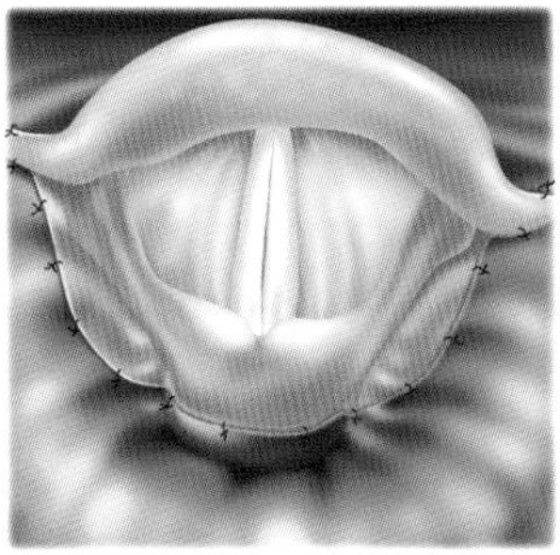

ENDOSCOPIC VIEW
By 6 months, both vocal folds had a midline position. The patients could speak during the occlusion of the tracheostomy.

Allotransplantation restricted to the larynx (1)

POTENTIAL CANDIDATES FOR LARYNGEAL TRANSPLANTATION INCLUDE APHONIC PATIENTS AFTER LARYNGEAL TRAUMA AND PATIENTS WITH LARGE BENIGN CHONDROMAS OR LOW-GRADE CHONDROSARCOMAS REQUIRING LARYNGECTOMY. AT PRESENT, BECAUSE OF THE INCREASED RISK OF A SECOND CANCER, PATIENTS WHO HAVE BEEN TREATED FOR LOCALLY ADVANCED OR RECURRENT THROAT CANCER SHOULD NOT BE CONSIDERED SUITABLE CANDIDATES.

The larynx can be transplanted on the superior thyroid and laryngeal vessels. We plan transplantation on both superior thyroid arteries and veins.

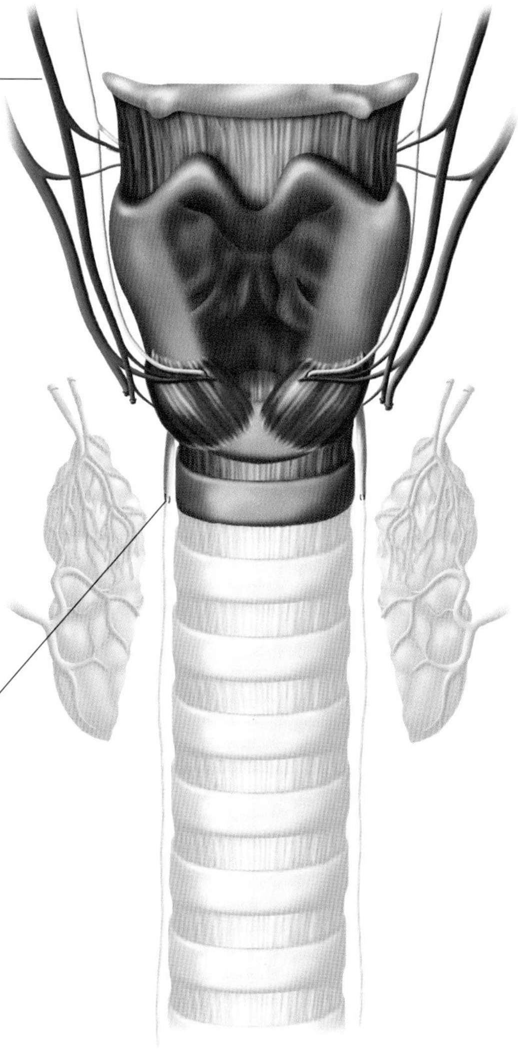

Our proposal for allotransplantation restricted to the larynx
Including the trachea and thyroid gland is not necessary in cases of laryngeal stenosis and chondrosarcomas restricted to the larynx. Including the cervical trachea and thyroid gland may augment morbidity in cases where the allotransplant needs removal because of complications.

Moreover, **recurrent nerve anastomosis** close to the larynx will be technically easier than an anastomosis that is low in the neck. The prognosis for motor reinnervation of the vocal folds may improve when the anastomosis is performed close to the end organ.

IN POTENTIAL CANDIDATES FOR LARYNGEAL TRANSPLANTATION, WE PROPOSE AN ADAPTED TRANSPLANTATION TECHNIQUE IN WHICH ONLY THE LARYNX IS TRANSPLANTED. THERE ARE SUFFICIENT SCIENTIFIC ARGUMENTS TO STATE THAT THIS ADAPTATION SHOULD LEAD TO LESS MORBIDITY AND COULD PROVIDE A GREATER CHANCE FOR THE SUCCESSFUL RE-INNERVATION OF THE VOCAL FOLDS. IT IS IMPORTANT TO NOTE THAT THERE IS AN ABSENCE OF MORBIDITY IN CASES OF TRANSPLANT FAILURE.

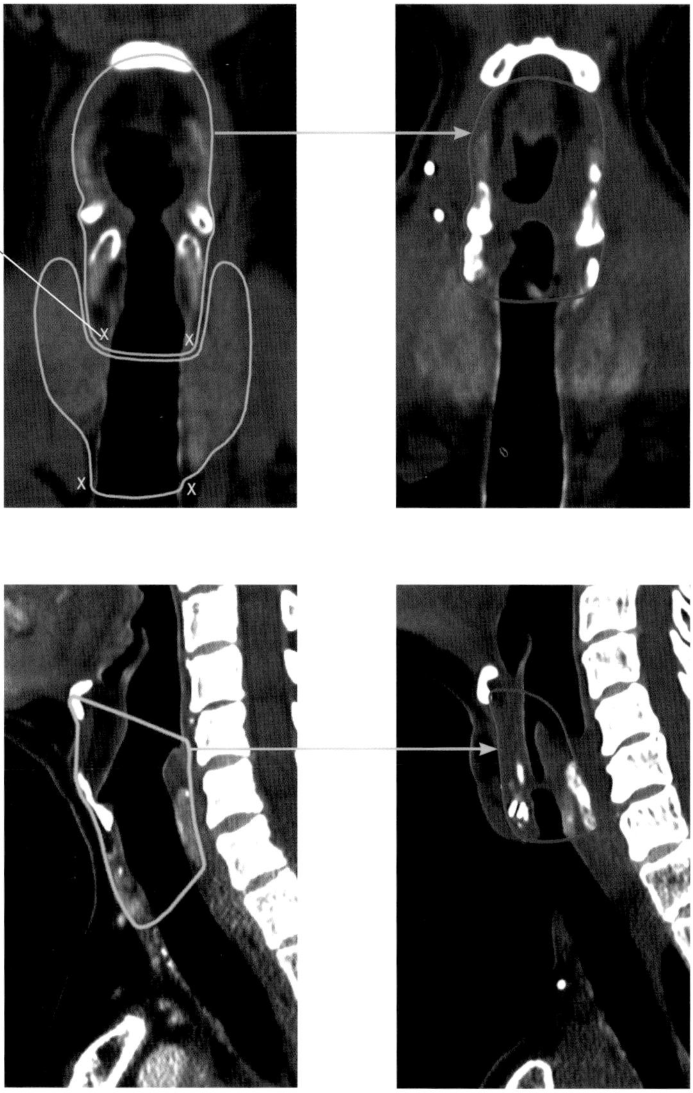
urrent
ngeal
ve
stomosis

A case of end-stage laryngeal stenosis

The patient is a 28-year-old woman with a completely stenotic larynx. She uses an external device (Electrolarynx) to speak. Her larynx is totally stenotic and shortened, with immobile arytenoid cartilages. We proposed to replace her stenotic larynx (red line) with a laryngeal allotransplant (blue line, blue arrow), but without including the trachea and thyroid gland (green line). She is currently waiting for a suitable allotransplant. The procedure is approved by the institutional review board of the University Hospitals Leuven, Belgium.

Allotransplantation restricted to the larynx (2)

THE MORE FAVORABLE REINNERVATION OF THE “LARYNX-ONLY” APPROACH MAY GIVE AN ADDITIONAL PROSPECT FOR VOCAL FOLD ABDUCTION, WHICH COULD LEAD TO CLOSURE OF THE TRACHEOSTOMY.

Proposal for allotransplantation restricted to the larynx
Nerve recovery is thought to take place at a rate of 1 mm a day from the point of traumatic injury. Nerve anastomosis immediately below the posterior cricoarytenoid muscle will be more favorable for successful reinnervation. There is only one muscle that causes laryngeal abduction and posterior motion of the arytenoids, namely the posterior cricoarytenoid muscle. The nerve anastomosis can be done immediately below the posterior cricoarytenoid muscle, which is much more favorable for successful reinnervation compared to anastomosis low inside the neck when the cervical trachea is included.

As inactive muscles atrophy over time, both the quality and the velocity of nerve regeneration are relevant in this context. Because the intelligibility and speech quality of an electrolarynx is lower than that of a voice prosthesis after laryngectomy, our patient with the complete laryngeal stenosis may well opt for total laryngectomy with a voice prosthesis placed in a tracheo-esophageal fistula. When the patient decides to undergo a total laryngectomy, selecting the ‘larynx-only transplantation option’ may become a logical choice. A larynx-only transplantation may improve her quality of life considerably. A new larynx with the vocal folds in the midline position that allows for the production of a relatively normal female voice would be considered successful.

The more favorable reinnervation of the larynx-only approach may give an additional prospect for vocal fold abduction, which could lead to closure of the tracheostomy. It is important to note that there is an absence of morbidity in cases of transplant failure. A status of total laryngectomy without additional mutilation will be obtained if the allotransplant requires removal because of complications related to the immunosuppressive medication or after complete transplant rejection.

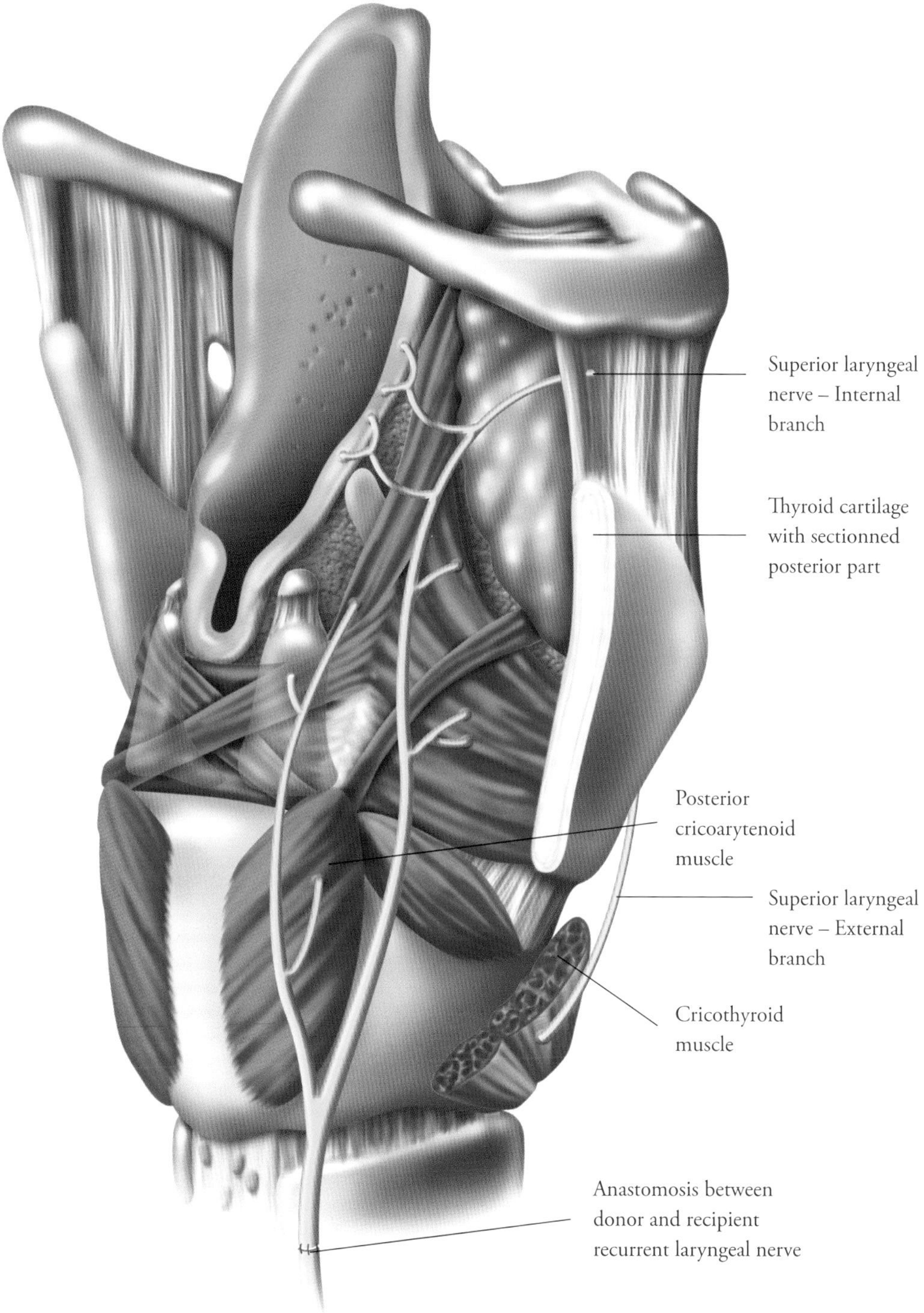
Superior laryngeal
nerve – Internal
branch
Thyroid cartilage
with sectionned
posterior part
Posterior
cricoarytenoid
muscle
Superior laryngeal
nerve – External
branch
Cricothyroid
muscle
Anastomosis between
donor and recipient
recurrent laryngeal nerve

Posterior laryngeal view
In the "larynx-only" approach, anastomosis of the recurrent laryngeal nerve can be performed immediately below the posterior cricoarytenoid muscle.

Using the plethora of images that Ervinck collects on his computer, he produces phantasmagoric images in what is effectively a creative interaction between his own imagination and the possibilities offered by digital media. His whole work seems to consist of an infinite number of elements that are playfully being de- and recomposed on a virtual playground.

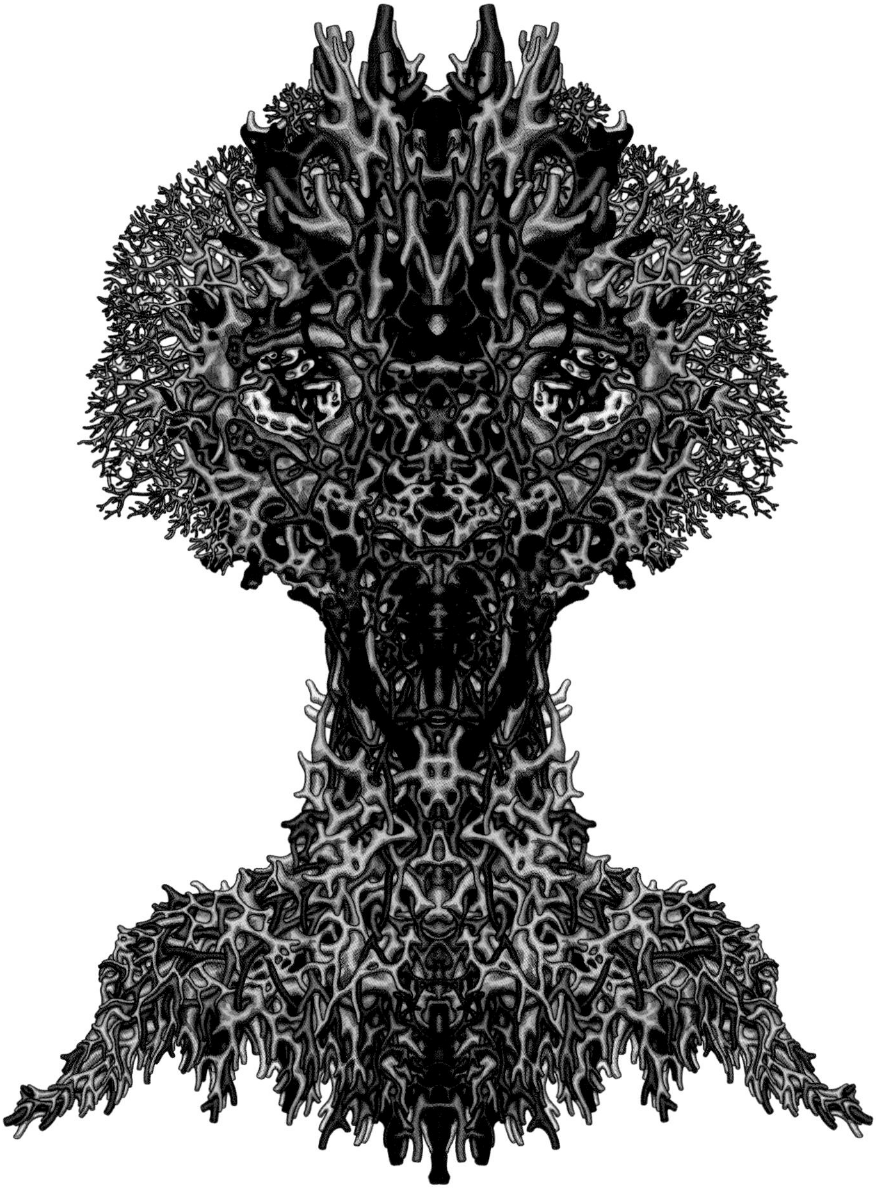

OCHIKORZ, 2010-2011

PRINT

155 × 120 CM

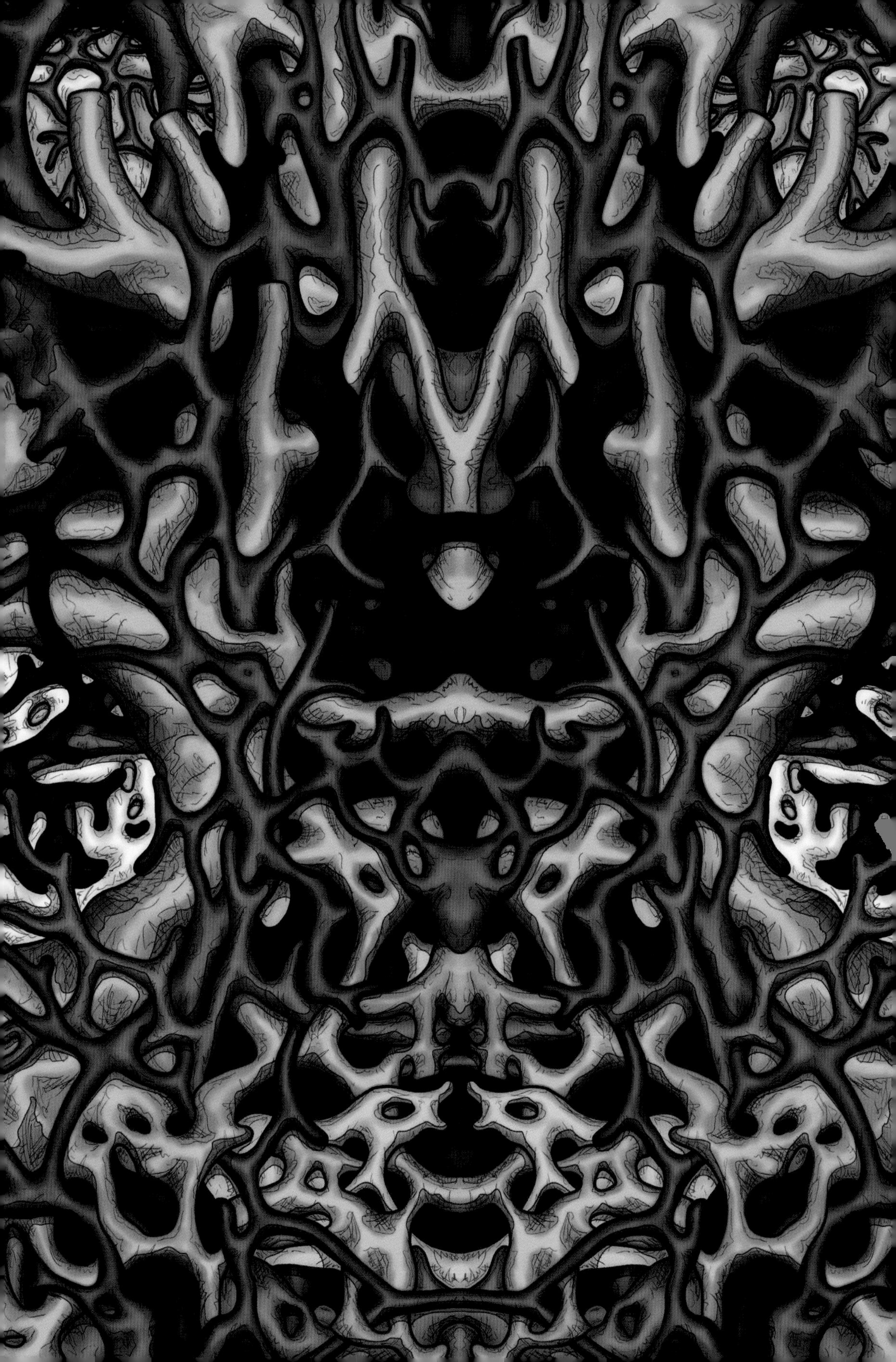

5. Laryngotracheal reconstruction with autologous tissue

Posterior glottic and subglottic stenosis (1) - (2)

Long-segment stenosis

Recurrent stenosis

A radial forearm flap lined with buccal mucosa can be used to resolve challenging cases of laryngeal, laryngotracheal and tracheal stenosis.

Posterior glottic and subglottic stenosis – (1)

USE OF REPAIR TISSUE WILL BE NECESSARY TO AUGMENT THE AIRWAY LUMEN AFTER THE INCISION AND EXPANSION OF THE STENOSIS. A FREE CARTILAGE GRAFT IS THE BEST OPTION TO HOLD THE POSTERIOR CRICOID INTO THE DISTRACTED POSITION. A CARTILAGE GRAFT CAN ALSO BE USED FOR THE AUGMENTATION OF THE ANTERIOR LARYNX AND THE ANTERIOR SUBGLOTTIC REGION. HOWEVER, THE HEALING OF CARTILAGE GRAFTS IS UNPREDICTABLE AND MAY RESULT IN NECROSIS. THE RECONSTRUCTED SITE IS STENTED FOR 4 TO 5 WEEKS.

RECONSTRUCTION

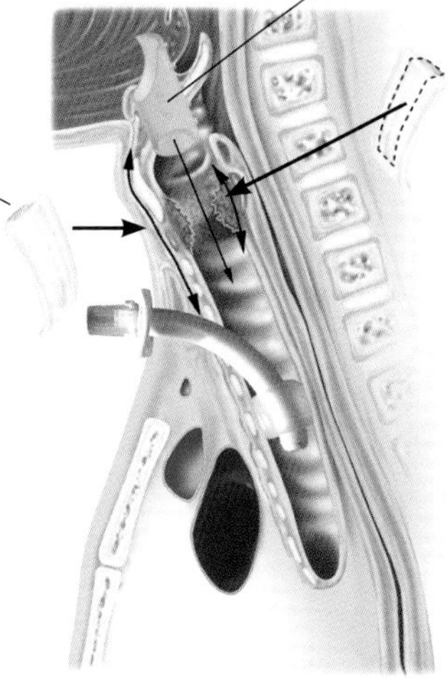
Silicone stent tailored to support the reconstruction
Anterior cartilage graft

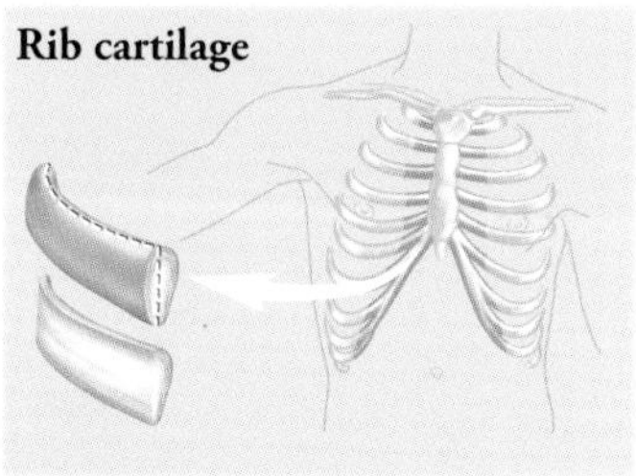
Rib cartilage

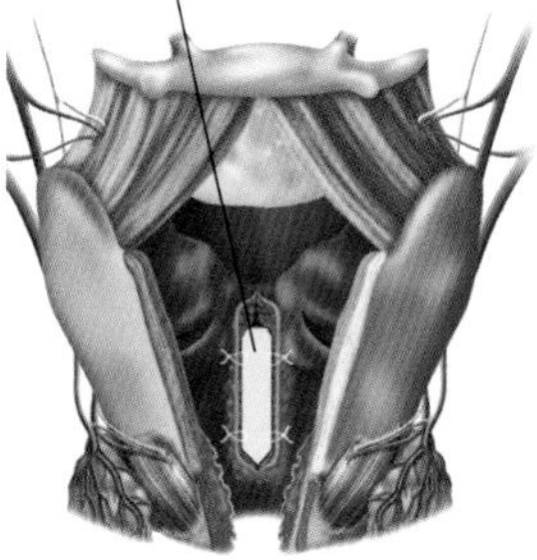
Posterior cartilage graft

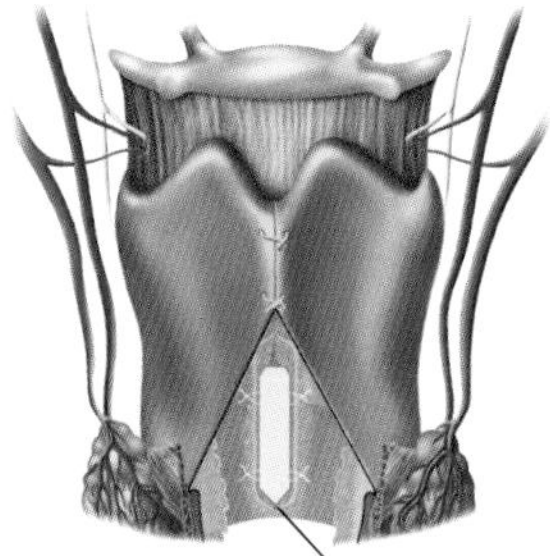
Anterior cartilage graft

Sagittal CT scan after reconstruction

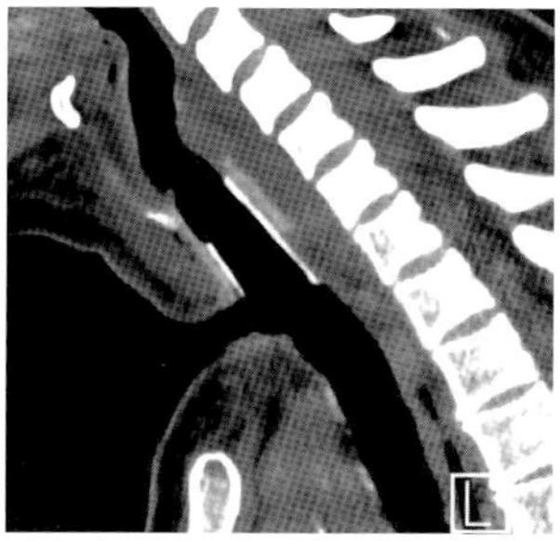

RECONSTRUCTIVE PROCEDURE

A costal cartilage graft is split in two parts. One part is sutured between the two distracted halves of the cricoid cartilage. A silicone stent is tailored to support the reconstruction and to stabilize the posterior cartilage graft during healing. The second part of the rib cartilage is used to close the anterior larynx. The stent is removed endoscopically after 1 month.

CARTILAGE GRAFTS

Although the cartilage grafts may show resorption (CT scan after 6 weeks), they are usually sufficient to resolve the posterior glottic stenosis with mild subglottic stenosis

BEFORE RECONSTRUCTION

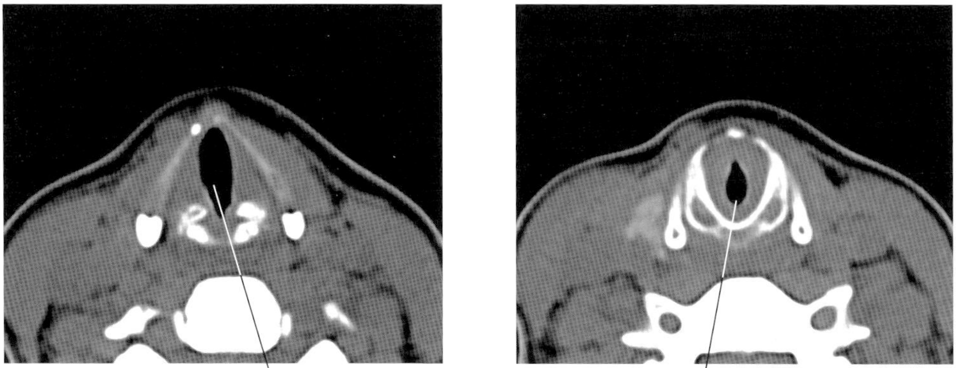
Posterior glottic stenosis
Mild subglottic stenosis

AFTER RECONSTRUCTION

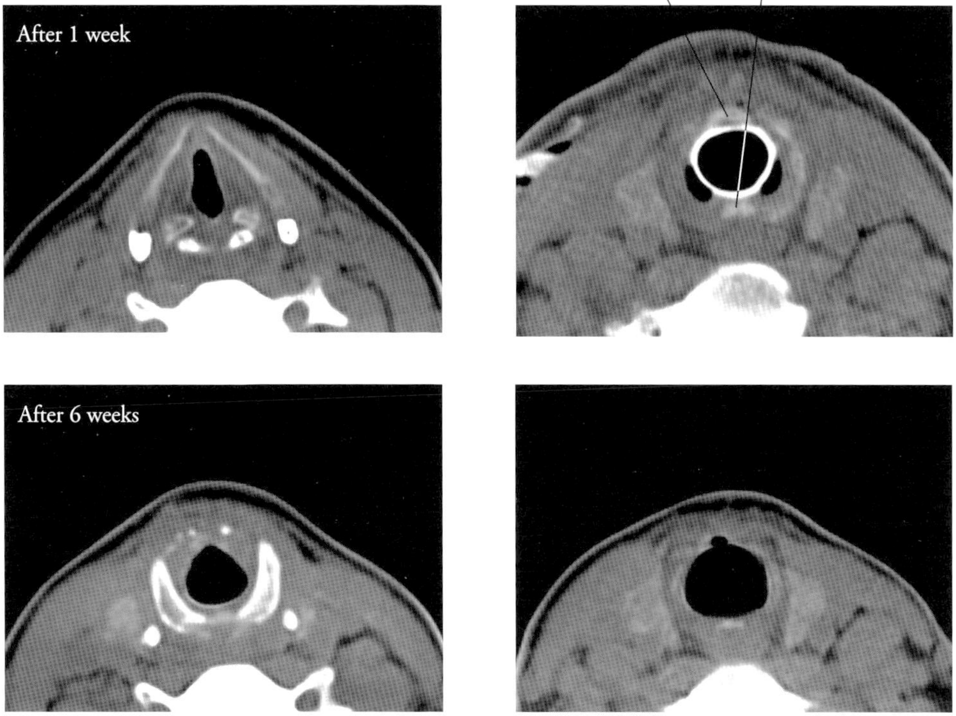
Anterior and posterior cartilage grafts
After 1 week
After 6 weeks

CT scan – axial section

Posterior glottic and subglottic stenosis – (2)

USE OF REPAIR TISSUE WILL BE NECESSARY TO AUGMENT THE AIRWAY LUMEN AFTER THE INCISION AND EXPANSION OF THE STENOSIS. A FREE CARTILAGE GRAFT IS THE BEST OPTION TO MAINTAIN THE POSTERIOR CRICOID IN THE DISTRACTED POSITION. TO GUARANTEE PRIMARY HEALING, A MUCOSAL-LINED FASCIAL FLAP MAY BE A BETTER CHOICE FOR AN ANTERIOR LARYNX RECONSTRUCTION IN CASES OF PRONOUNCED STENOSIS ANTERIORLY. THE RECONSTRUCTED SITE IS STENTED FOR 4 TO 5 WEEKS.

RECONSTRUCTION

The silicone stent is tailored to support the reconstruction.

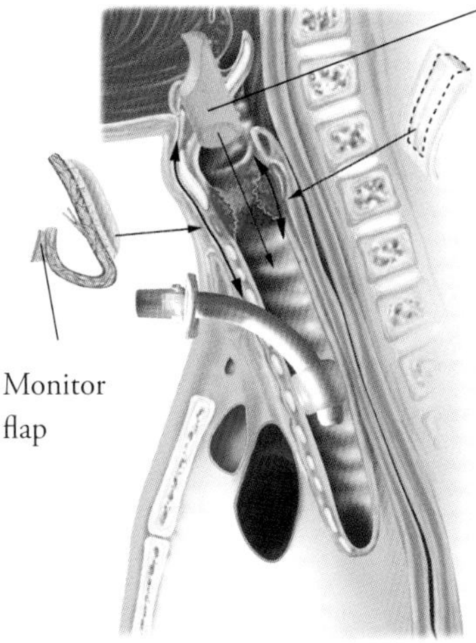

Monitor flap

RECONSTRUCTIVE PROCEDURE

A costal cartilage graft is sutured between the two distracted halves of the cricoid cartilage. The mucosal-lined fascia is sutured to the anterior defect. A silicone stent is tailored to support the reconstruction and to stabilize the posterior cartilage graft during healing. The radial blood vessels are anastomosed to the neck vessels (superior thyroid artery and internal jugular vein). The stent is removed endoscopically after 1 month.

Pronounced anterior part of stenosis.

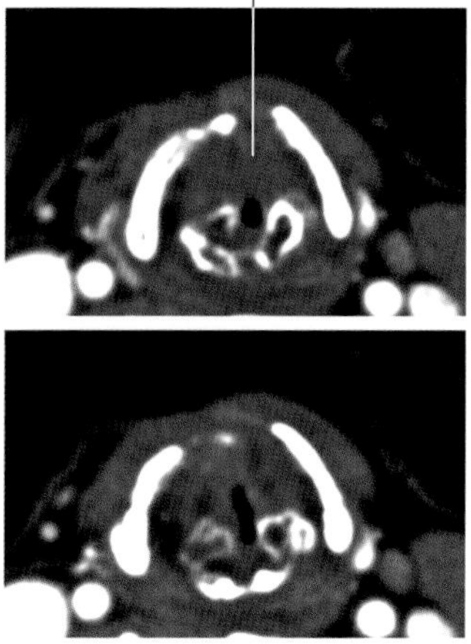

Preoperative CT scan – Axial view

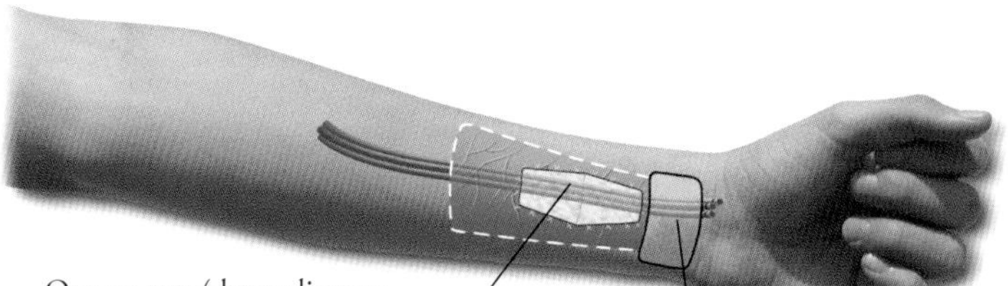

One or two (depending on the size of the defect) buccal mucosal grafts (approximately 1.2 cm width and 1.5 cm long) are sutured (Vicryl 5.0) to the radial forearm fascia.

The skin paddle will serve as a monitor flap.

AFTER RECONSTRUCTION

Sagittal view

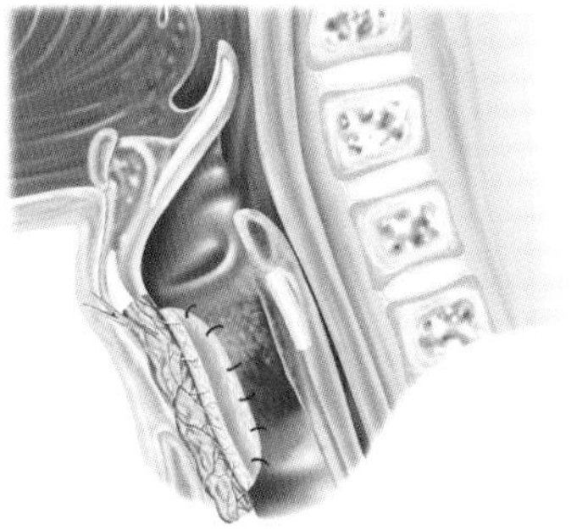

The mucosal graft is visible at the glottic and subglottic level.

Endoscopic view anteriorly

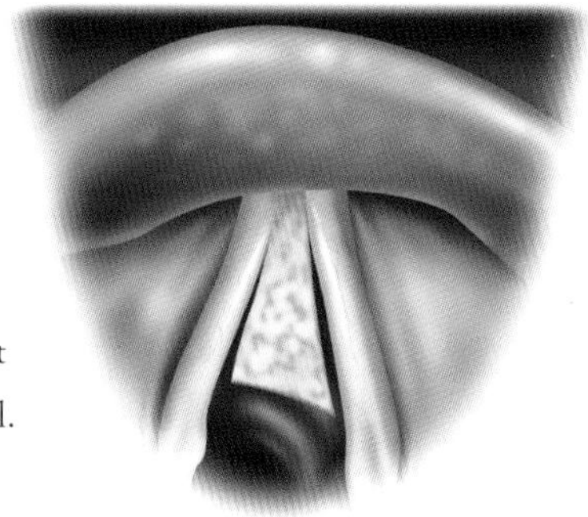

> "The healing of avascular cartilage is unpredictable; it is, however, the only tissue that can be placed in the posterior larynx."
>
> "In the anterior larynx, mucosal-lined fascia is preferred because it guarantees primary healing."

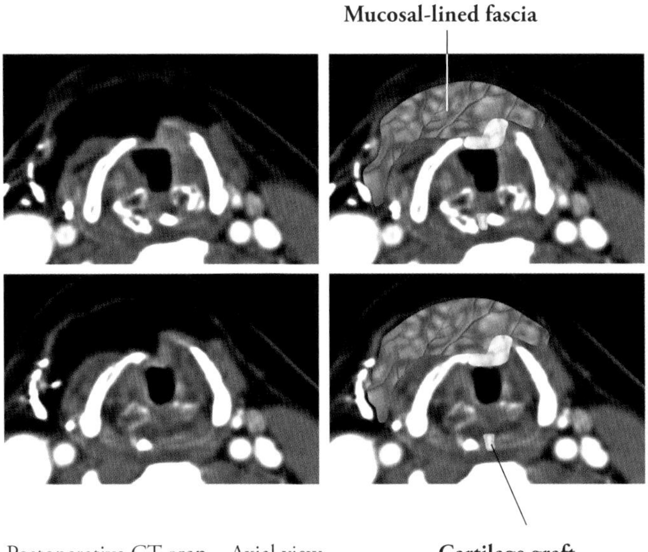
Mucosal-lined fascia
Cartilage graft

Postoperative CT scan – Axial view

Long-segment stenosis

SOME LONG SEGMENT STENOSES MAY BE SUITABLE FOR A LONGITUDINAL INCISION, EXPANSION, AND PLACEMENT OF A MUCOSAL-LINED FASCIAL FLAP.

A **Dumon stent** is made of silicone with regularly placed external studs to help anchor it to the tracheal wall. The **stent** is available in a variety of diameters (6 to 18 mm) and lengths (20 to 80 mm).

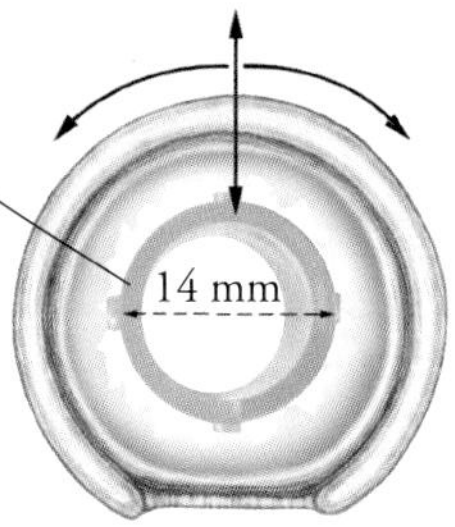
14 mm

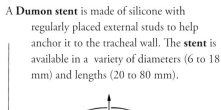

The **stent** is fixed with Vicryl sutures so that the external studs can be removed.

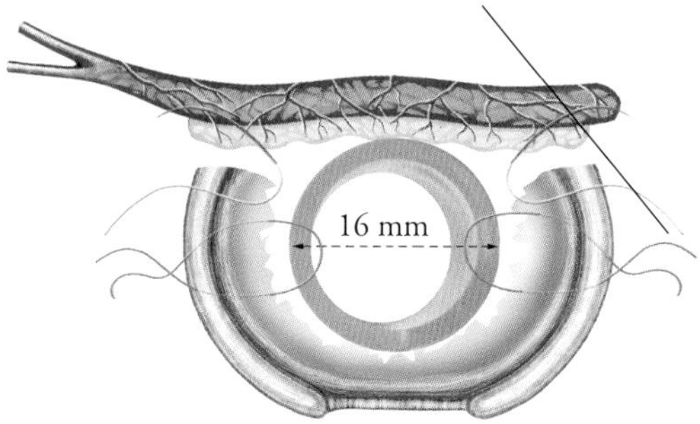
16 mm

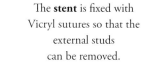

CT scan – coronal section

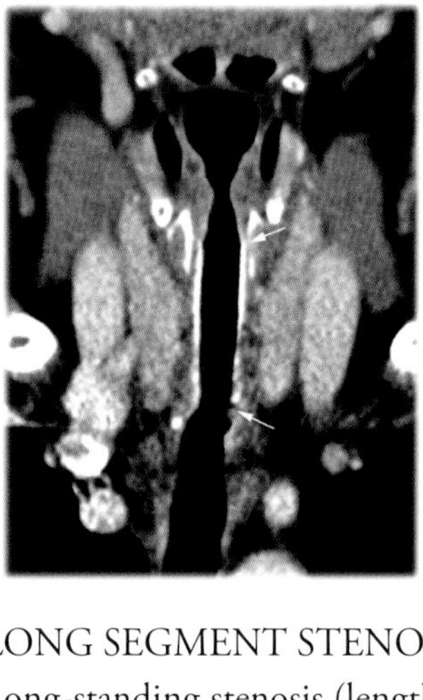

Sagittal view

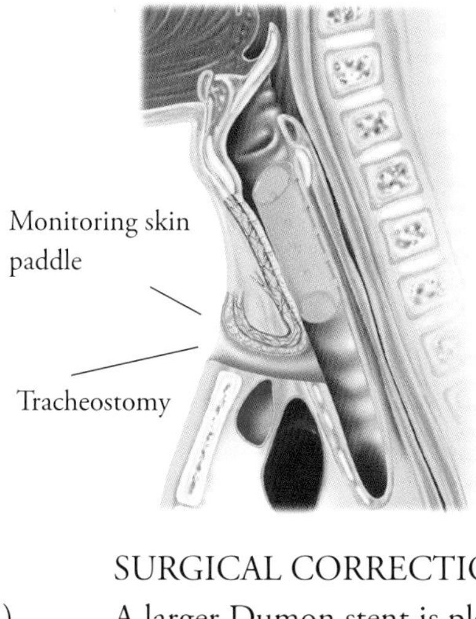
Monitoring skin paddle
Tracheostomy

LONG SEGMENT STENOSIS

Long-standing stenosis (length, 6 cm) of the subglottic region and the cervical trachea (postintubation). A Dumon silicone stent (between white arrows) has been placed to support the airway temporarily. The stenosis is incised longitudinally (double arrow) and expanded (black arrows).

SURGICAL CORRECTION

A larger Dumon stent is placed in the expanded airway. The anterior airway defect is reconstructed with the mucosal-lined fascia. A tracheostomy is placed below the reconstruction. The stent can be removed via rigid bronchoscopy.

THIS RECONSTRUCTION CAN BE USED TO RESTORE THE LONG ANTERIOR AIRWAY DEFECT WITH SUFFICIENT REMAINING NATIVE AIRWAY CONCAVITY.

REPAIR TISSUE

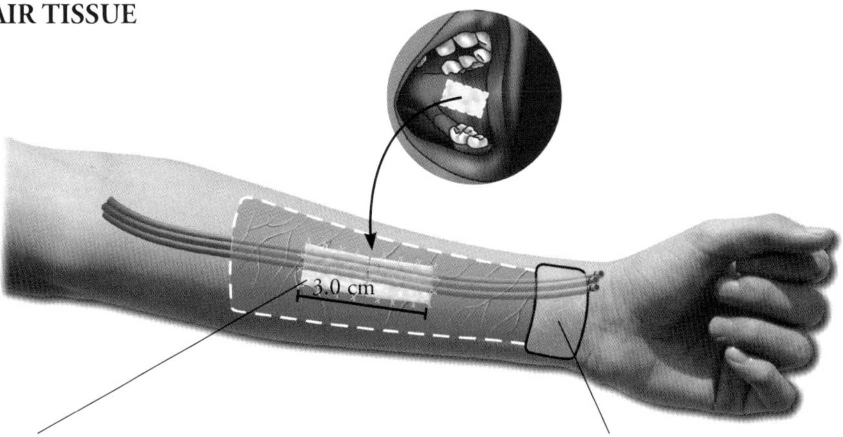
3.0 cm

Two **full-thickness buccal mucosa grafts** (about 1.2 by 3.0 cm) are sutured to the fascia flap.

Monitoring skin paddle

SITUATION AFTER RECONSTRUCTION

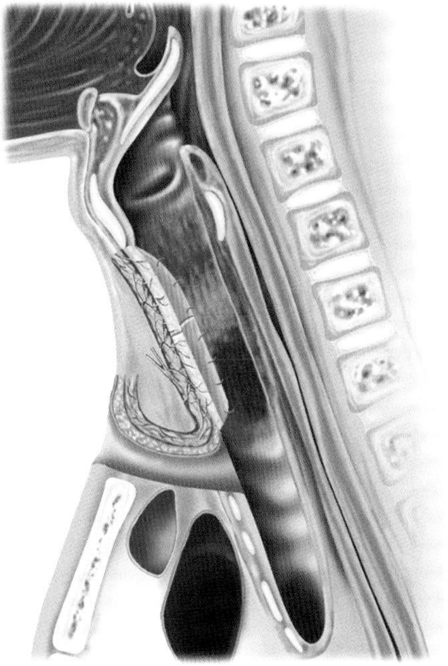

Sagittal view after stent removal (after 4-5 weeks)

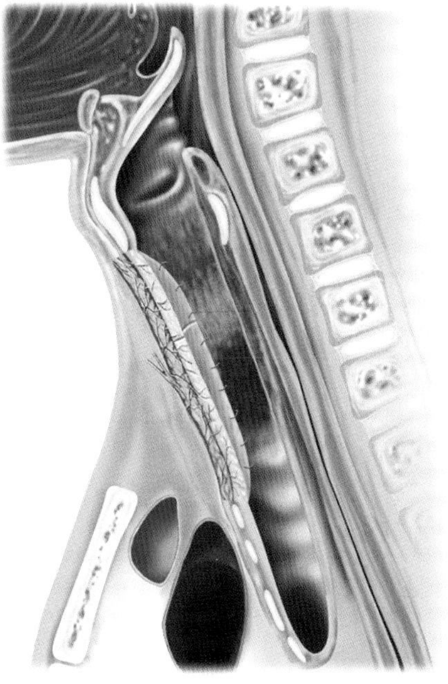

Sagittal view after closure of the tracheostomy

Recurrent stenosis

A MUCOSAL-LINED RADIAL FOREARM FASCIA FLAP IS OUR PREFERRED AUTOLOGOUS TISSUE RECONSTRUCTION TECHNIQUE AFTER THE INCISION AND EXPANSION OF THE RECURRENT STENOSIS AFTER SEGMENTAL RESECTION.

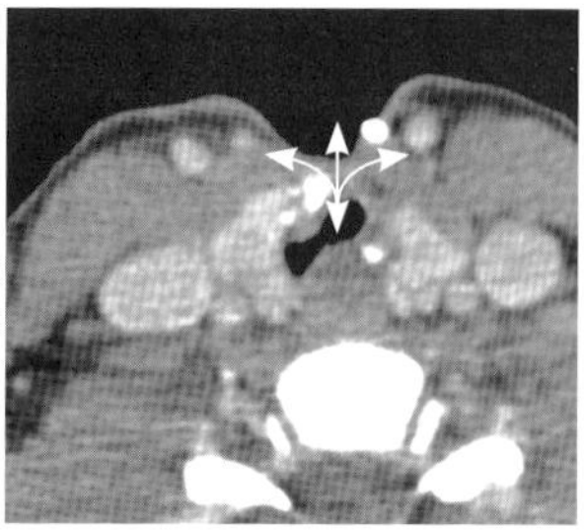

CT scan – axial section

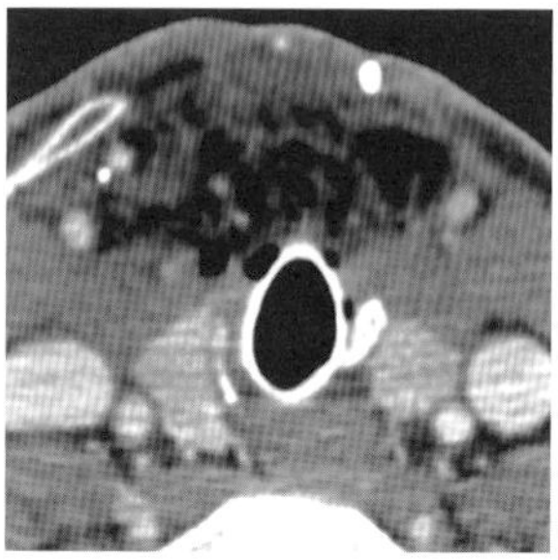

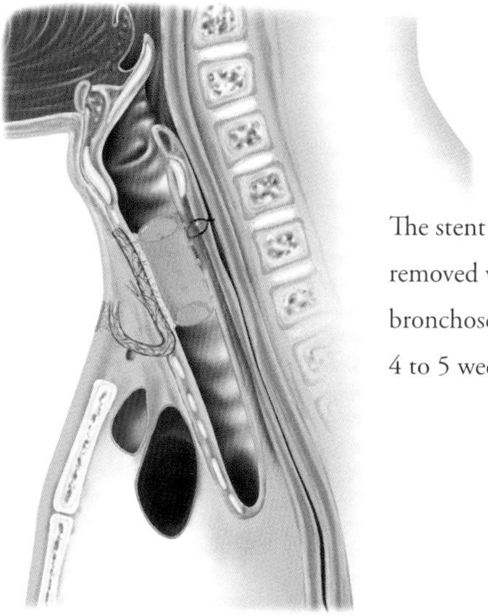

The stent can be removed with rigid bronchoscopy after 4 to 5 weeks.

CT scan – sagittal section

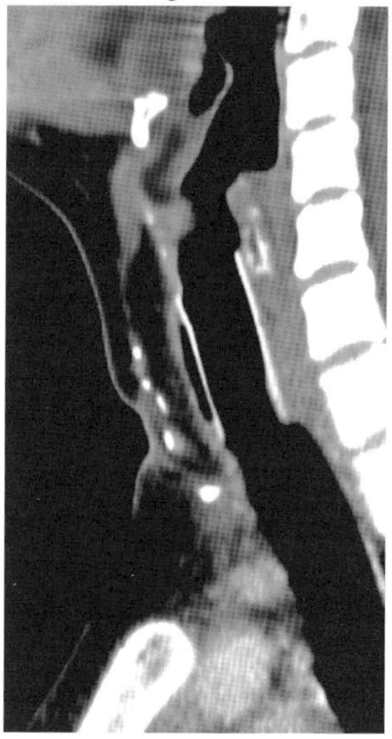

CT scan after reconstruction with a **silicone stent** supporting the reconstruction.

CORRECTION OF THE RE-STENOSIS

A re-stenosis at the anastomosis after segmental resection is incised anteriorly (double arrow) and expanded (arrows). A mucosal-lined radial forearm fascial flap is sutured into the airway defect. A silicone stent will support the reconstructed airway during 4-5 weeks. The stent is secured with one or two Vicryl sutures (3.0 or 2.0) to prevent migration.

MORPHOLOGY AFTER RECONSTRUCTION

The stent can be removed with rigid bronchoscopy after 4-5 weeks. The anterior tracheal defect is repaired with a mucosal-lined (between arrows) radial forearm fascial flap. Sufficient airway concavity remains from the native airway (double arrow).

Axial view

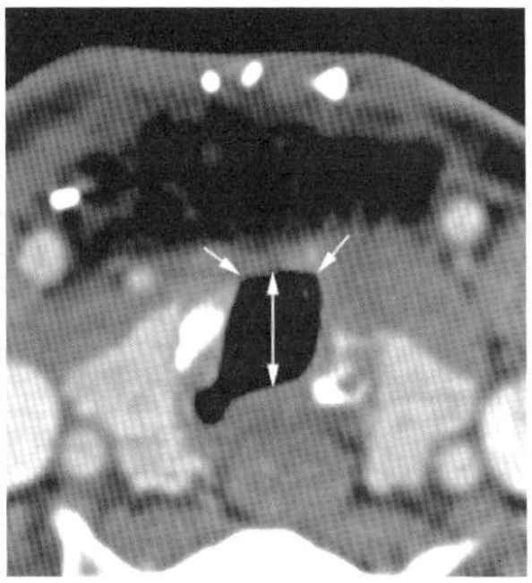

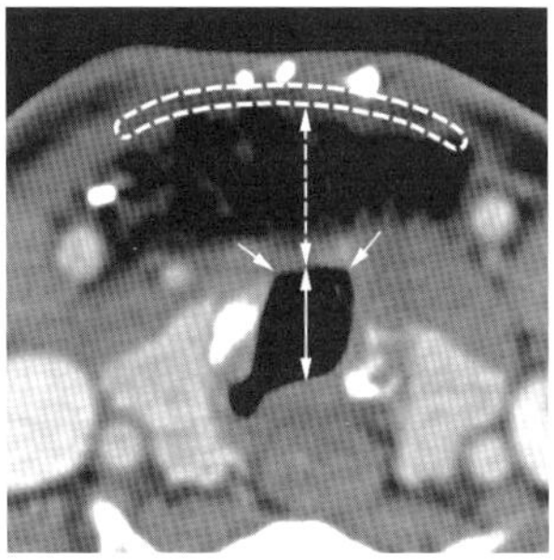

Adding **rigid material** (dotted line) to the soft tissue reconstruction would not bring improvements to the supportive value of the reconstruction because of the thickness of the soft tissue flap (dotted double arrow).

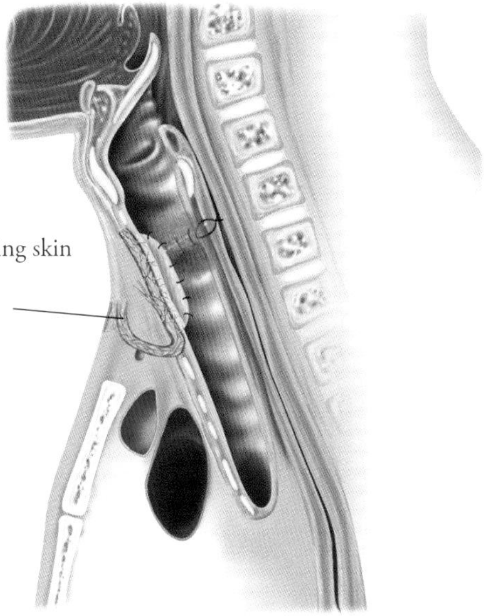
Monitoring skin paddle

Situation after stent removal

"A mucosal-lined radial fascial flap will repair the anterior airway defect linearly."

Ervinck's compositions are indefinable, originating from elongated forms and so-called blobs that structure the resulting three-dimensional organic form. Using 'copy paste', he applies images, shapes and textures of extremely diverse origins.

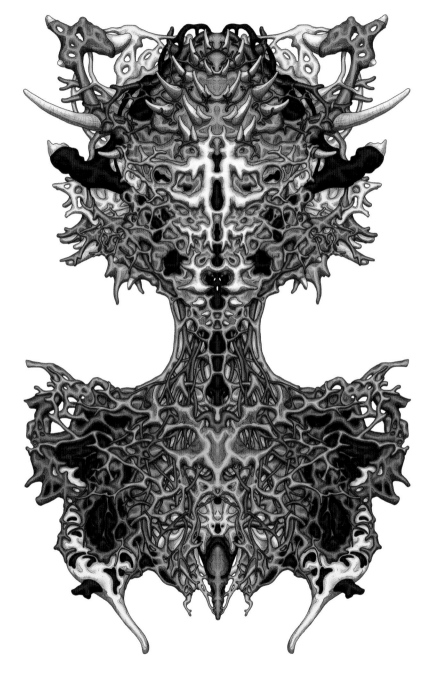

EDNIRIAORZ, 2010-2011

PRINT

155 × 120 CM

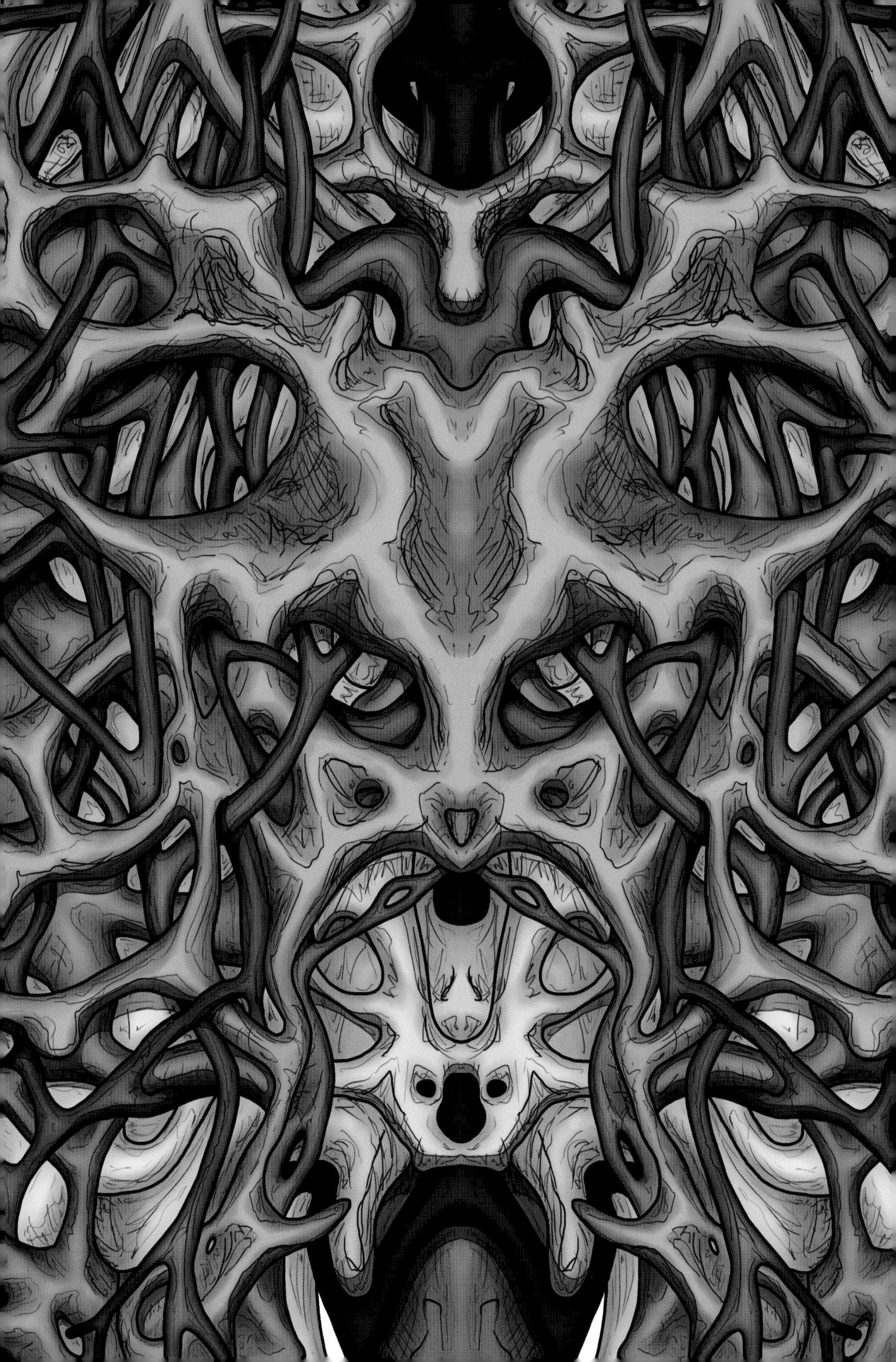

6. Tracheal allotransplantation – background

Experimental allograft revascularization

Heterotopic revascularization

Experimental orthotopic transplantation

Experimental rejection

Rejection and anastomotic repopulation

Rejection and repopulation of the graft midportion

Vascular induction versus angiogenesis

We started experimental animal research on tracheal allotransplantation in 1995. With the exception of some anecdotal, poorly documented cases (without blood supply restoration or immunosuppressive medication), no clinical tracheal allotransplants were orthotopically transplanted as an isolated composite tissue transplant. One paper was published that reported a successful heterotopic tracheal revascularization in the abdomen of an immunosuppressed recipient.

Experimental allograft revascularization

TRACHEAL ALLOTRANSPLANTS CAN BECOME REVASCULARIZED IN THE HETEROTOPIC POSITION. IN IMMUNOSUPPRESSED RABBITS, THE RECIPIENT BLOOD SUPPLY OF THE FASCIAL FLAP WILL INDUCE REVASCULARIZATION AND MUCOSAL REGENERATION OVER A 14-DAY PERIOD.

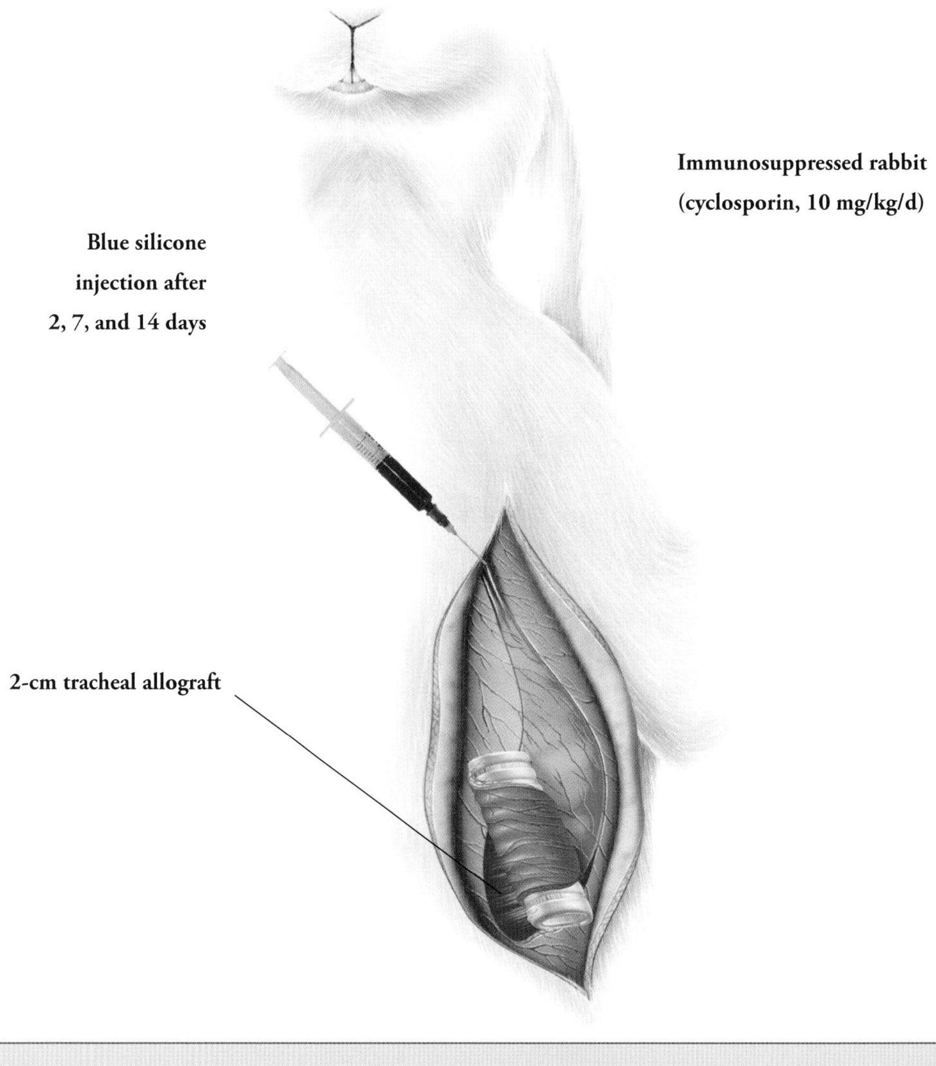
Immunosuppressed rabbit
(cyclosporin, 10 mg/kg/d)
Blue silicone
injection after
2, 7, and 14 days
2-cm tracheal allograft

"Tissue regeneration refers to the replacement of lost or damaged tissue with an 'exact' copy, such that both morphology and functionality are completely restored".

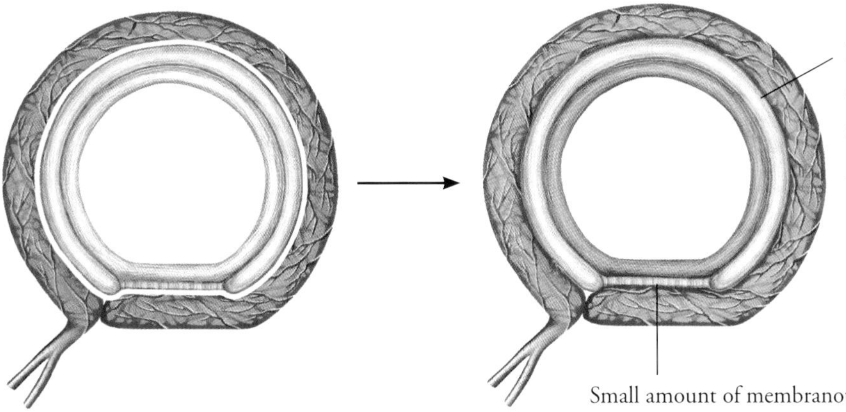
DAY 1
DAY 14
In rabbits, the cartilaginous trachea forms a nearly circular ring.
Small amount of membranous trachea

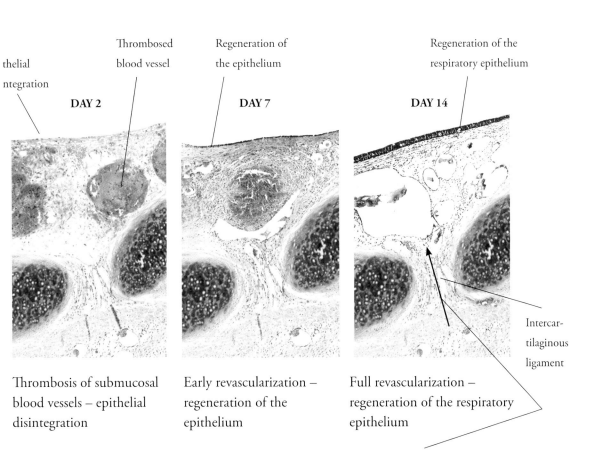

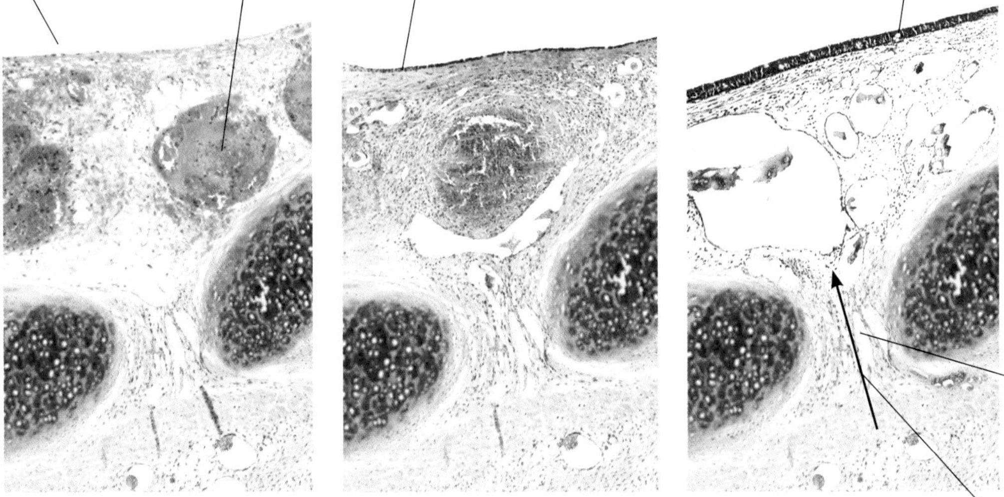
thelial
ntegration
Thrombosed blood vessel
Regeneration of the epithelium
Regeneration of the respiratory epithelium
DAY 2
DAY 7
DAY 14
Intercar-tilaginous ligament

Thrombosis of submucosal blood vessels – epithelial disintegration

Early revascularization – regeneration of the epithelium

Full revascularization – regeneration of the respiratory epithelium

Vascular induction from the surrounding fascia during initial revascularization

Heterotopic revascularization

THE OMENTUM HAS BEEN USED IN INDIRECT TRACHEAL REVASCULARIZATION. IN HUMANS, A SINGLE CASE REPORT HAS BEEN PUBLISHED ON HETEROTOPIC TRACHEAL REVASCULARIZATION BY OMENTUM WRAPPING IN THE ABDOMINAL POSITION (KLEPETKO ET AL., J THORAC CARDIOVASC SURG, 2004; 127: 862-867.). IN THIS REPORT, A 57-YEAR-OLD MALE PATIENT WITH TERMINAL CHRONIC PULMONARY DISEASE WAS PLANNED TO UNDERGO LUNG TRANSPLANTATION. HE HAD A HISTORY OF MULTIPLE EPISODES OF RESPIRATORY FAILURE, WHICH HAD RESULTED IN THE REPEATED NEED FOR MECHANICAL VENTILATION AND TRACHEOSTOMIES. TRACHEAL STENOSIS HAD DEVELOPED AS A CONSEQUENCE OF

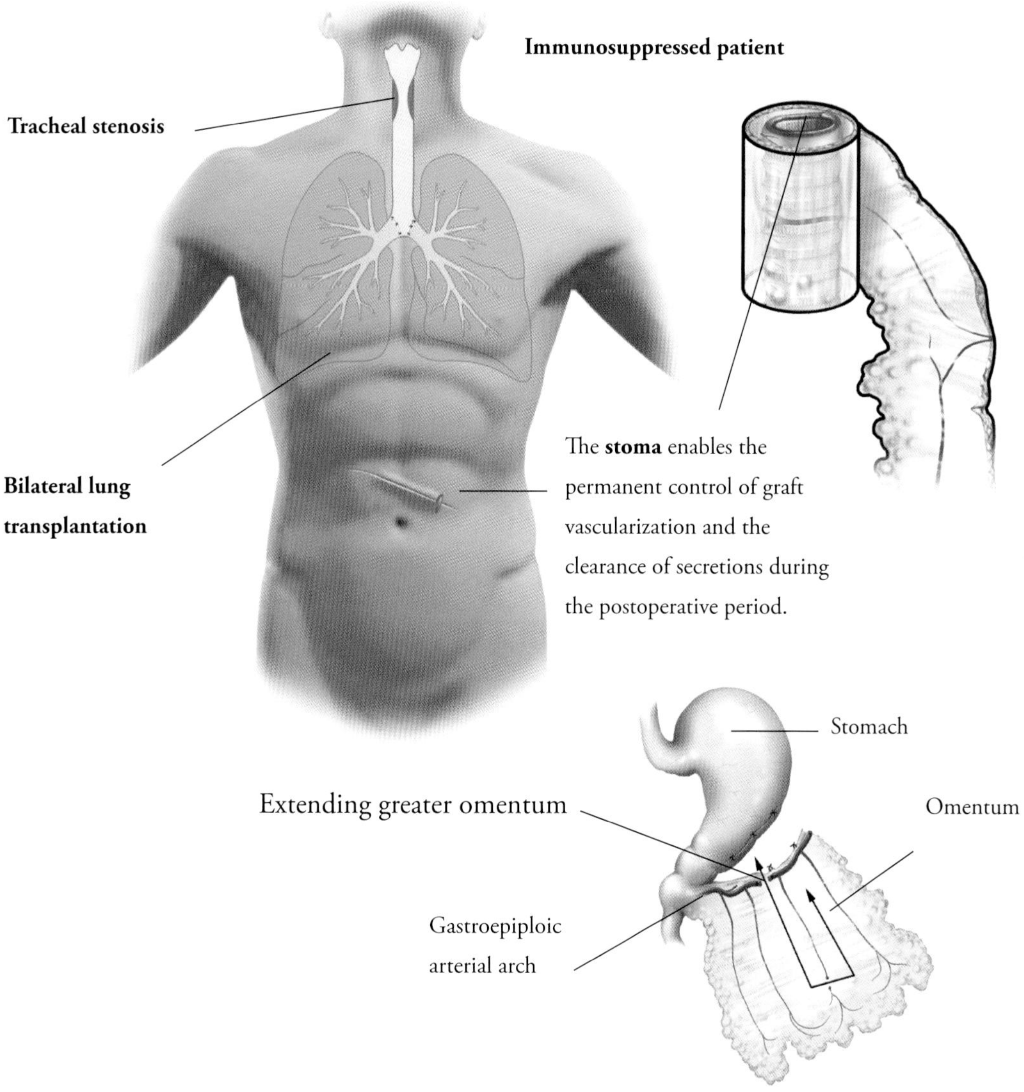
Immunosuppressed patient
Tracheal stenosis
Bilateral lung transplantation
The stoma enables the permanent control of graft vascularization and the clearance of secretions during the postoperative period.
Stomach
Extending greater omentum
Omentum
Gastroepiploic arterial arch

THESE INTERVENTIONS. THE PATIENT WAS OFFERED A STAGED PROCEDURE, WHICH CONSISTED OF A BILATERAL LUNG TRANSPLANTATION WITH THE TRANSFER OF THE DONOR TRACHEA INTO THE RECIPIENT'S ABDOMEN, WRAPPED IN THE GREATER OMENTUM. THIS LEFT THE OPTION FOR A LATER RESECTION OF THE STENOTIC TRACHEAL SEGMENT FOLLOWED BY A RECONSTRUCTION WITH THE TRACHEAL ALLOTRANSPLANT THAT HAD BEEN REVASCULARIZED AND PEDICLED FROM THE OMENTUM.

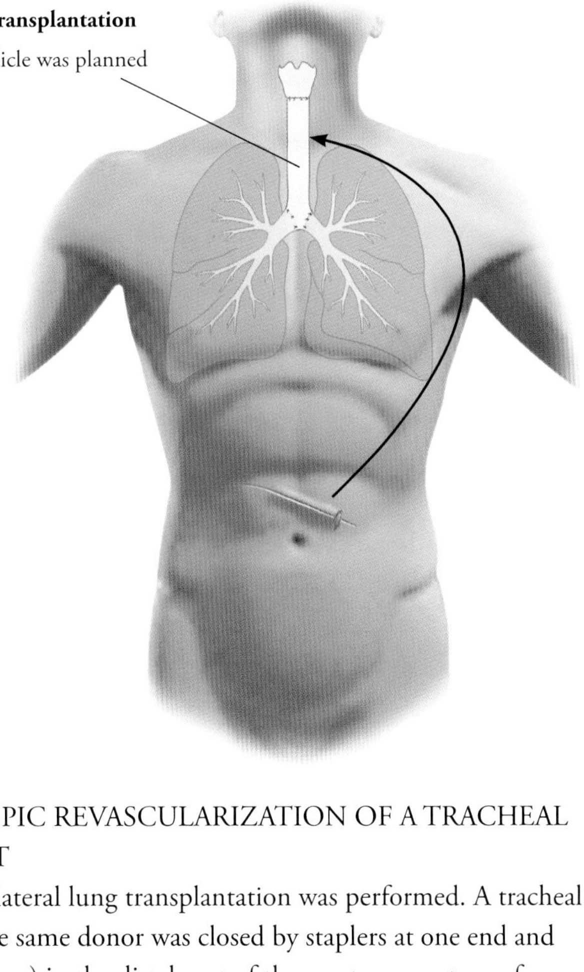

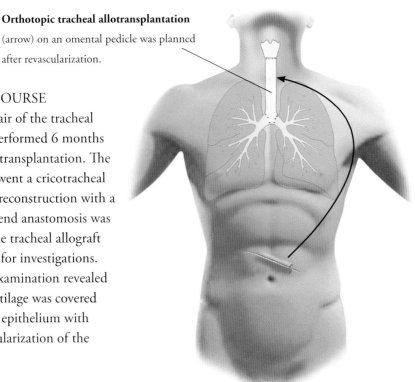

Orthotopic tracheal allotransplantation (arrow) on an omental pedicle was planned after revascularization.

CLINICAL COURSE

Definitive repair of the tracheal stenosis was performed 6 months after the lung transplantation. The patient underwent a cricotracheal resection and reconstruction with a direct end-to-end anastomosis was achievable. The tracheal allograft was harvested for investigations. Histological examination revealed that viable cartilage was covered by respiratory epithelium with excellent vascularization of the tracheal wall.

HETEROTOPIC REVASCULARIZATION OF A TRACHEAL ALLOGRAFT

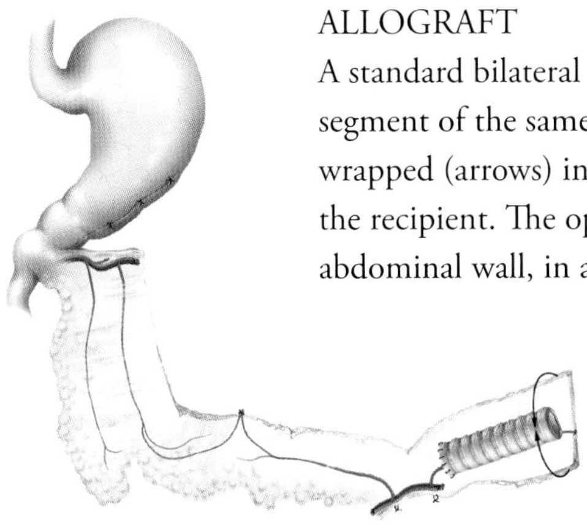

A standard bilateral lung transplantation was performed. A tracheal segment of the same donor was closed by staplers at one end and wrapped (arrows) in the distal part of the greater omentum of the recipient. The open end of the trachea was sutured into the abdominal wall, in a similar manner to a stoma.

Experimental orthotopic transplantation

RABBIT TRACHEAL ALLOGRAFTS UNDER CONTINUOUS IMMUNOSUPPRESSION WITH CYCLOSPORIN (10 MG/KG/DAY) SHOWED NO REJECTION. AFTER A 14-DAY REVASCULARIZATION PERIOD IN THE HETEROTOPIC POSITION, THE ALLOGRAFT COULD BE TRANSPLANTED ORTHOTOPICALLY ON THE NEWLY CREATED VASCULAR PEDICLE OF THE FASCIAL FLAP.

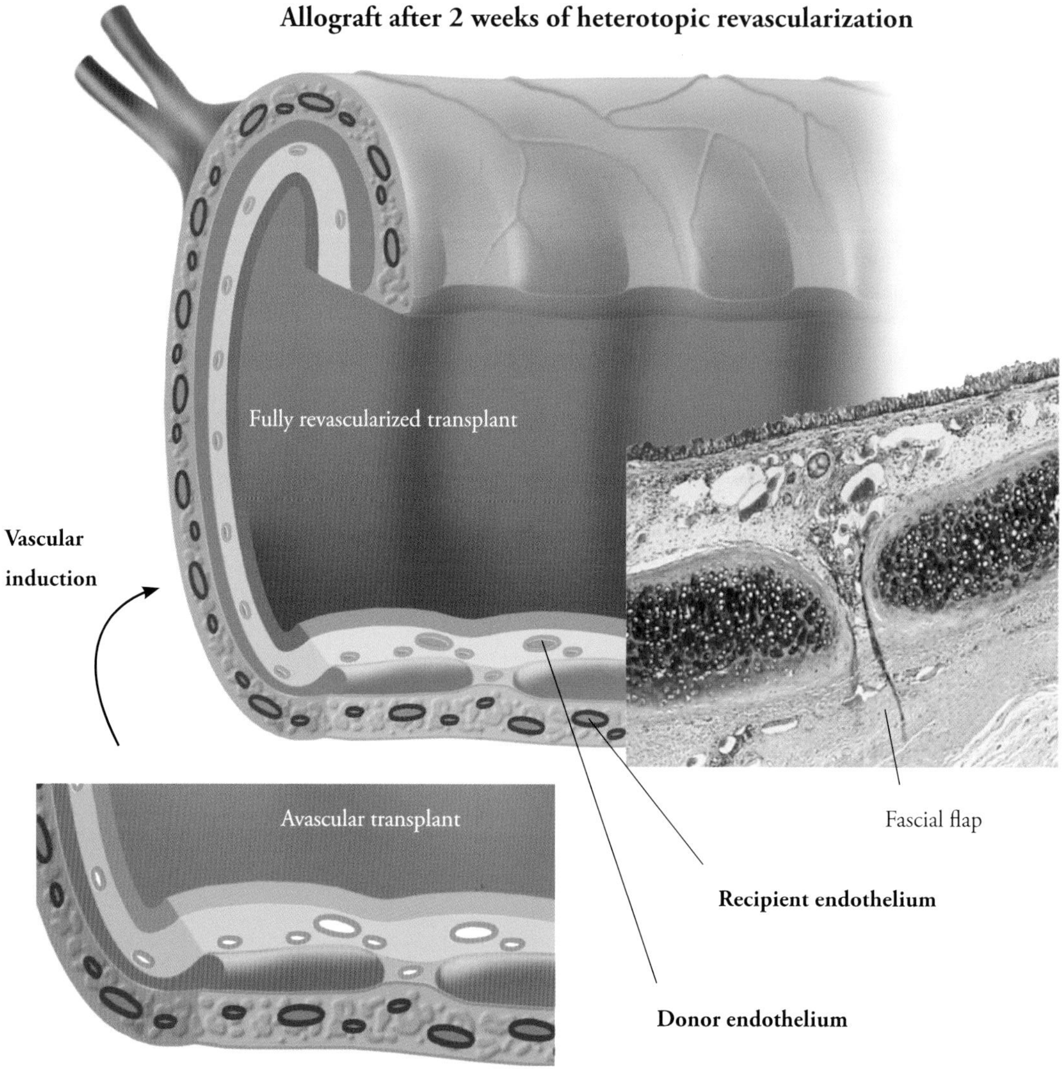
Allograft after 2 weeks of heterotopic revascularization
Fully revascularized transplant
Vascular induction
Avascular transplant
Fascial flap
Recipient endothelium
Donor endothelium

"Immunosuppressive medication preserves the morphologic and functional integrity of the tracheal allotransplant".

Orthotopic tracheal allotransplant in the immunosuppressed rabbit
Allogaft after 4 weeks of orthotopic transplantation under protection of immunosuppressive medication.

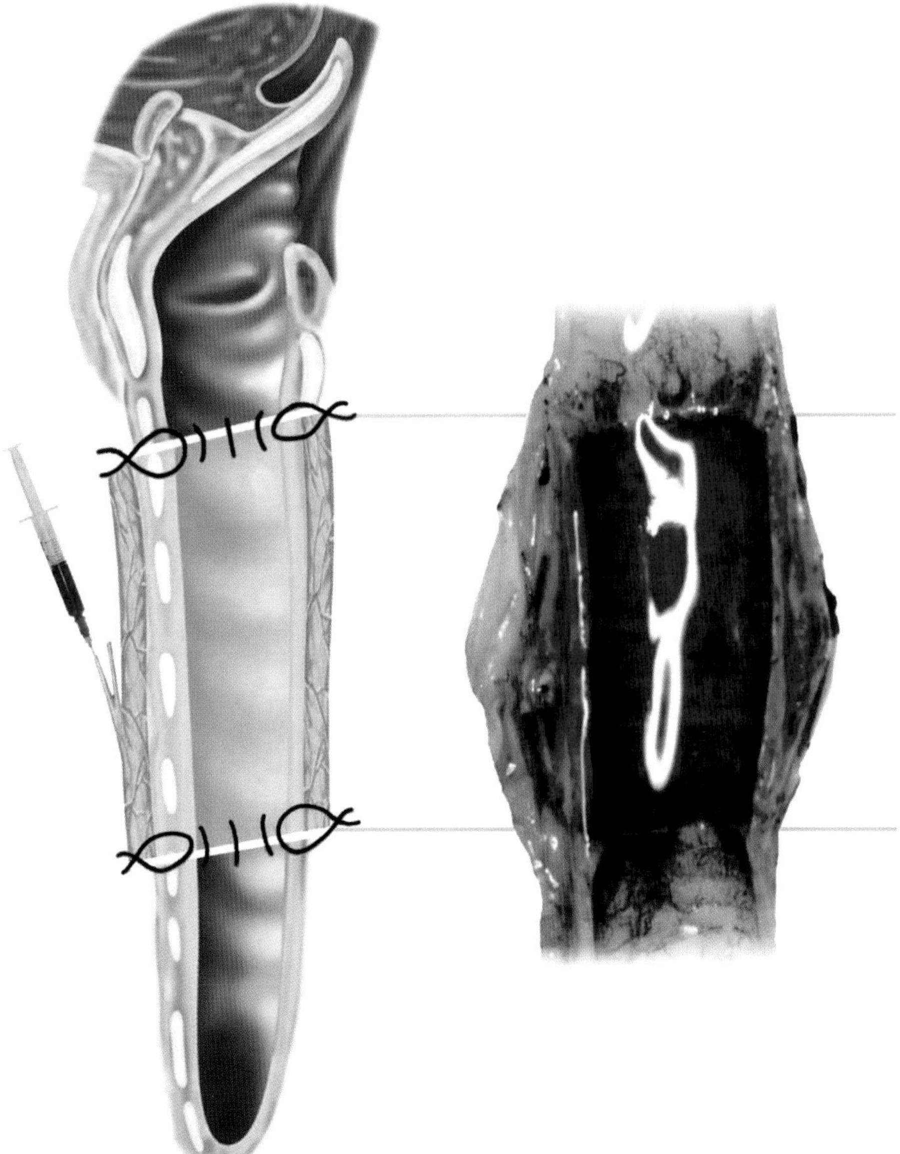

POSTMORTEM MACROSCOPY OF THE TRACHEAL ALLOGRAFT
The vascular pedicle of the fascia flap was injected with blue silicone and the trachea was incised posteriorly. Fascia and mucosal lining of the tracheal transplant were uniformly colored by blue silicone dye.

Experimental rejection

AFTER ORTHOTOPIC TRACHEAL ALLOTRANSPLANTATION, ACUTE REJECTION RESULTED AFTER THE CESSATION OF SHORT-TERM (4-5 WEEKS) IMMUNOSUPPRESSIVE MEDICATION.

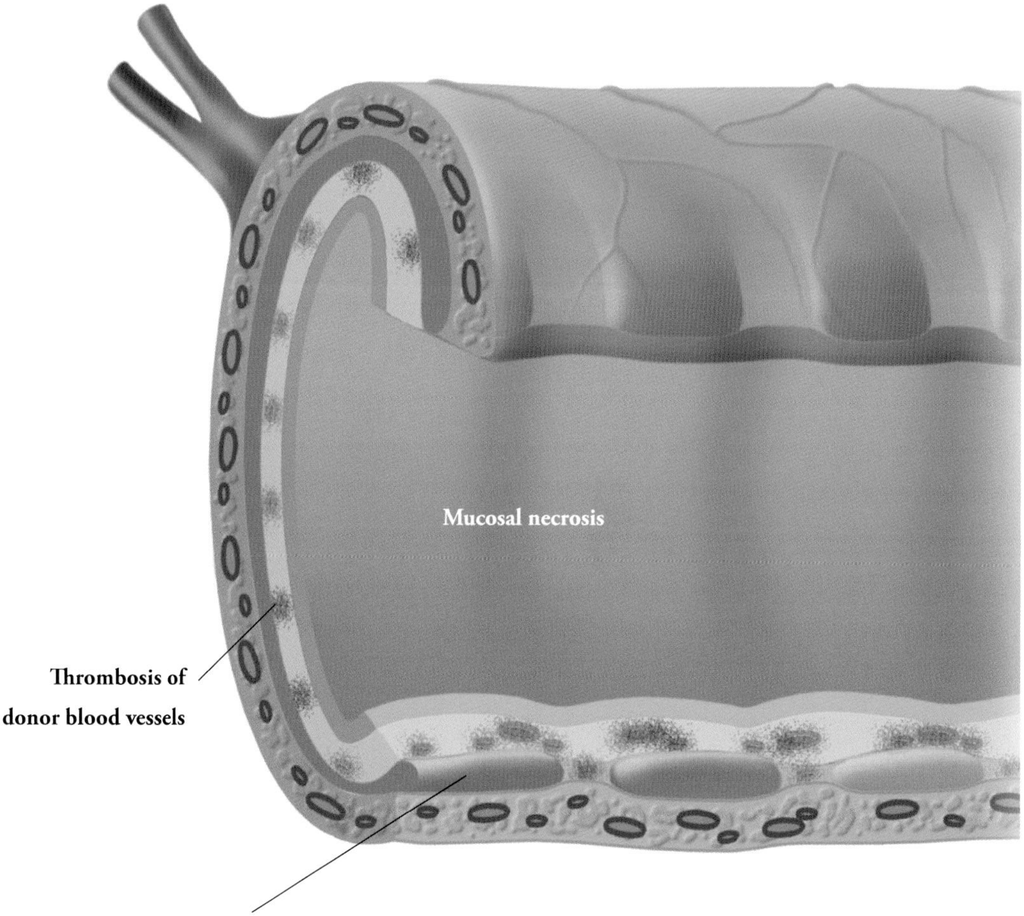
Mucosal necrosis
Thrombosis of
donor blood vessels

Cartilage is an avascular structure with chondrocytes protected within a matrix. Cartilage preserves its viability through diffusion from the surrounding vascularized tissues. The cartilage was not rejected directly by the immune system, but underwent secondary necrosis after the rejection-induced necrosis of the mucosal lining.

Intact recipient endothelium

ACUTE REJECTION

Immunologically-induced lymphocytes attack the microcirculation of the transplant. Rejection leads to thrombosis of the donor-derived blood vessels and to necrosis of the mucosal layer. Respiratory distress follows an average of **10 days after the abrupt cessation of short-term (4-5 weeks)** immunosuppressive treatment.

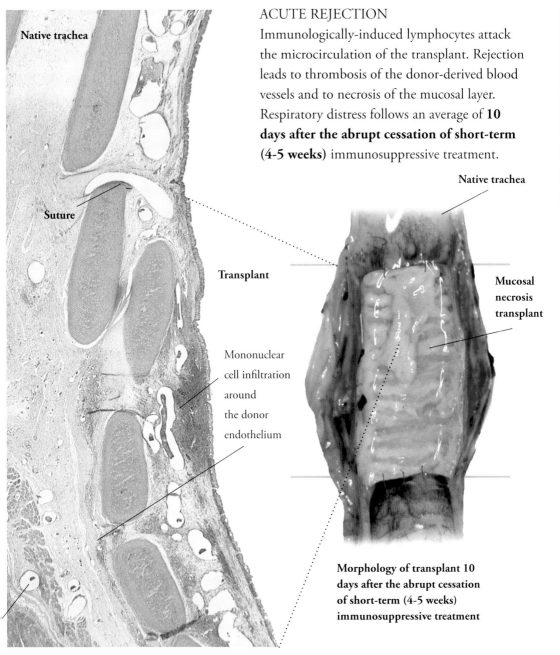

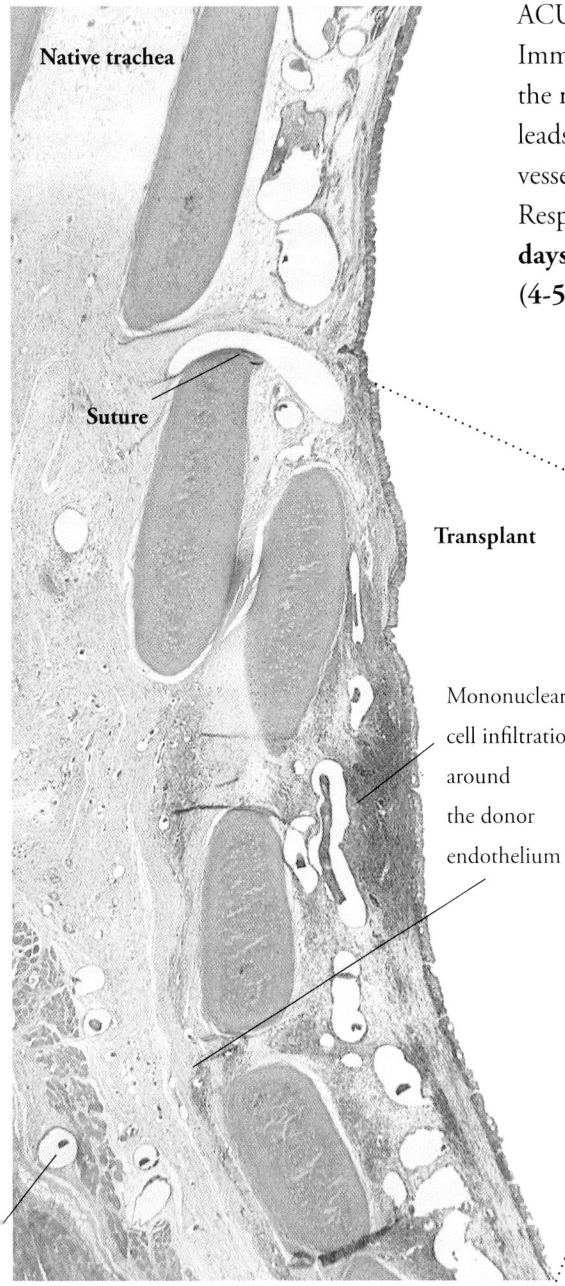
Native trachea
Suture
Transplant
Mononuclear cell infiltration around the donor endothelium

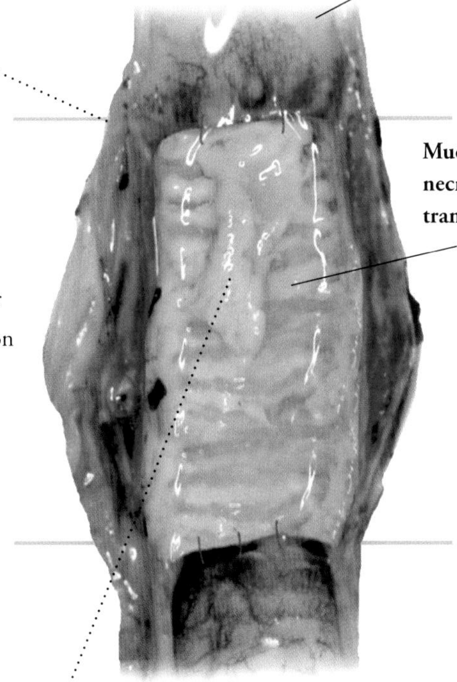
Native trachea
Mucosal necrosis transplant

Morphology of transplant 10 days after the abrupt cessation of short-term (4-5 weeks) immunosuppressive treatment

Histology of transplant 8 days after the abrupt cessation of short-term (4-5 weeks) immunosuppressive treatment

"The trachea is an organ subject to the same immunologic laws as all other allogenic tissues: the most important component in tracheal rejection is cell-mediated and the prime target cell population is allograft endothelium".

Rejection and anastomotic repopulation

CHRONIC REJECTION STUDIES IN RABBITS WERE PERFORMED TO EVALUATE THE POSSIBILITY OF THE WITHDRAWAL OF LONG-TERM IMMUNOSUPPRESSIVE MEDICATION. CHRONIC REJECTION WAS STUDIED WHEN IMMUNOSUPPRESION WAS STOPPED PROGRESSIVELY AFTER A RELATIVELY LONG PERIOD (4-5 MONTHS) OF IMMUNOSUPPRESSION.

CHRONIC REJECTION

These studies provided evidence for the possibility of tracheal allotransplant endothelial and epithelial repopulation from the native trachea (arrows). The repopulation capacity of the native trachea is length-dependent and confined to the anastomotic regions. This process is characterized by true angiogenesis with recipient capillary sprouts advancing across the graft-host junction with vascular reperfusion of the chronically rejected submucosal layer. The midportion of the transplant underwent necrosis because the intercartilaginous ligaments served as an obstruction to the ingrowth of recipient blood vessels. Respiratory distress follows after an average period of 4 weeks and after gradual withdrawal of long-term (4-5 months) immunosuppressive medication.

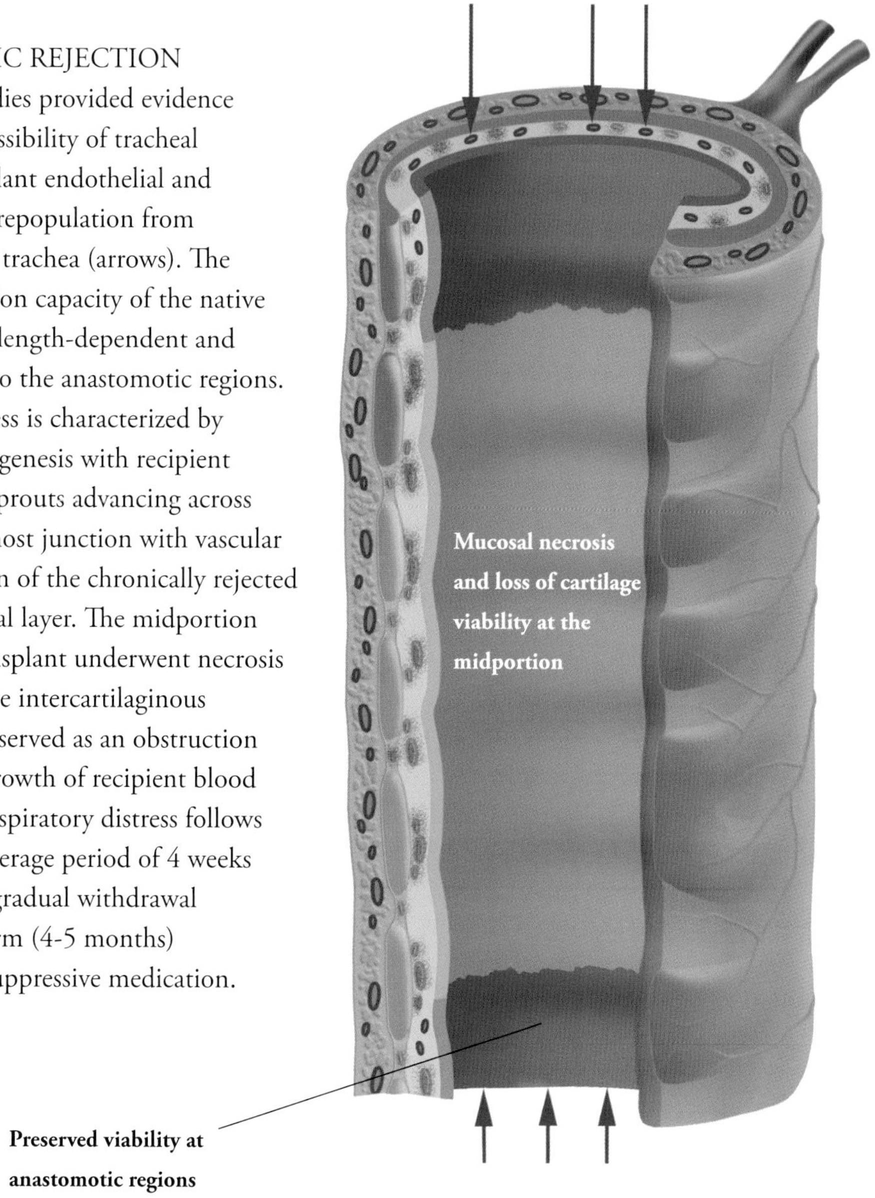
Mucosal necrosis and loss of cartilage viability at the midportion
Preserved viability at anastomotic regions

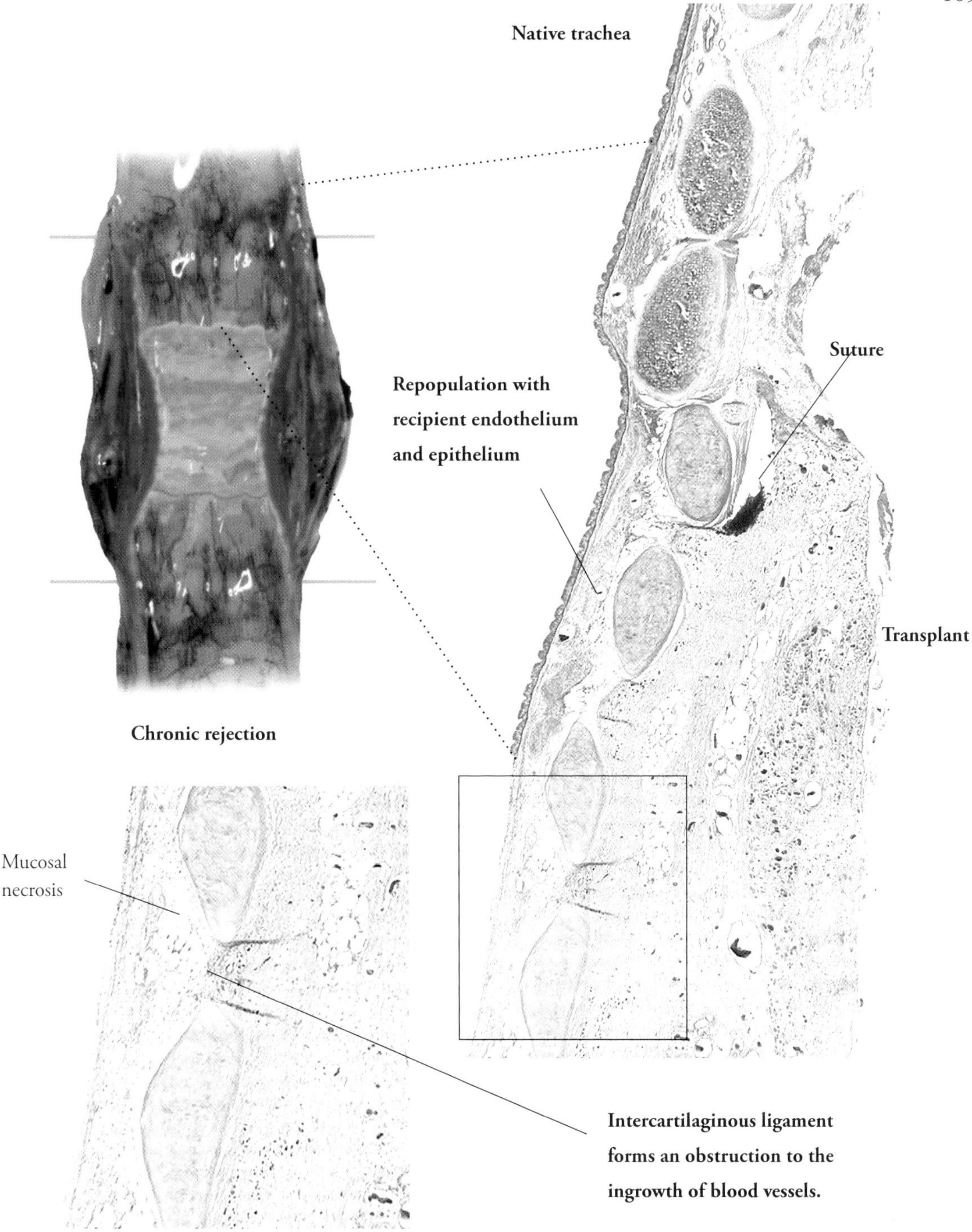
Native trachea
Suture
Repopulation with
recipient endothelium
and epithelium
Transplant
Chronic rejection
Mucosal
necrosis
Intercartilaginous ligament
forms an obstruction to the
ingrowth of blood vessels.

"Vascular induction and true angiogenesis are two different processes: vascular induction occurs through the intercartilaginous ligaments whereas these ligaments form an obstruction for the ingrowth of recipient blood vessels".

Vascular induction versus angiogenesis

VASCULAR INDUCTION IS THE REPERFUSION OF AN ALREADY ESTABLISHED VASCULAR NETWORK. THE RECIPIENT BLOOD VESSELS WILL REPERFUSE THE DONOR SUBMUCOSAL BLOOD VESSELS IN A HETEROTOPIC POSITION.

Avascular donor mucosa at time of implantation

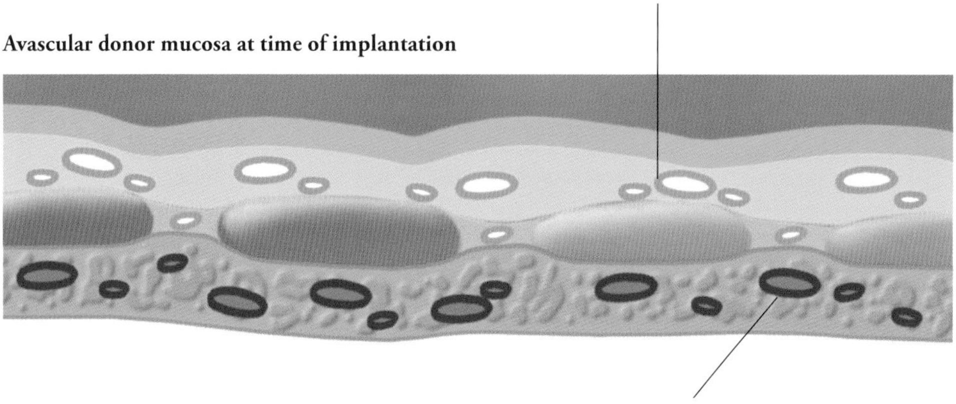
Donor endothelium
Recipient endothelium

Revascularized donor mucosa

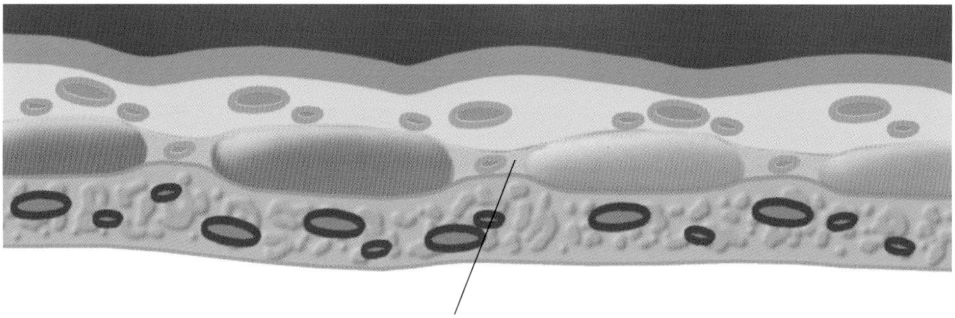
Vascular induction can occur through an intact intercartilaginous ligament.

ANGIOGENESIS IS THE PROCESS INVOLVING THE GROWTH OF NEW BLOOD VESSELS. RECIPIENT CAPILLARY SPROUTS CAN ADVANCE ACROSS THE GRAFT-HOST JUNCTION ONLY AT THE SITES WHERE THE INTERCARTILAGINOUS LIGAMENTS ARE INTERRUPTED. ANGIOGENESIS MAY LEAD TO VASCULAR REPERFUSION OF THE CHRONICALLY REJECTED SUBMUCOSAL LAYER.

Chronically rejected mucosal lining

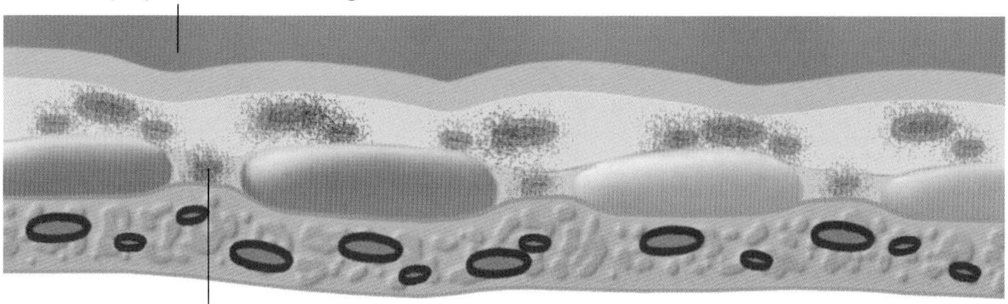

Intercartilaginous ligament forms an obstruction to angiogenesis.

Incisions of the intercartilaginous ligaments at time of implantation

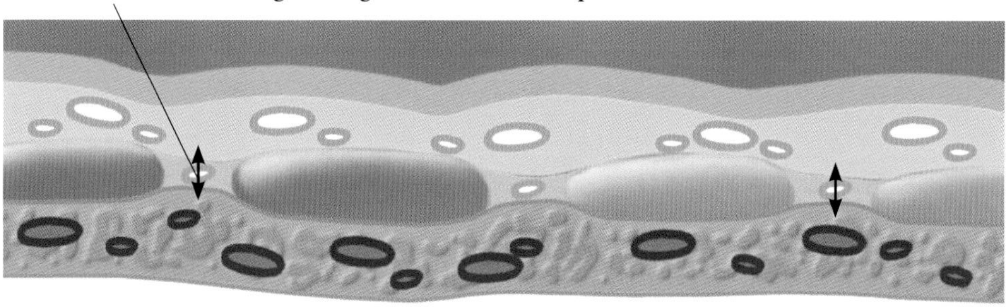

The recipient endothelial cells of the induced vascular nerwork are resistant to rejection

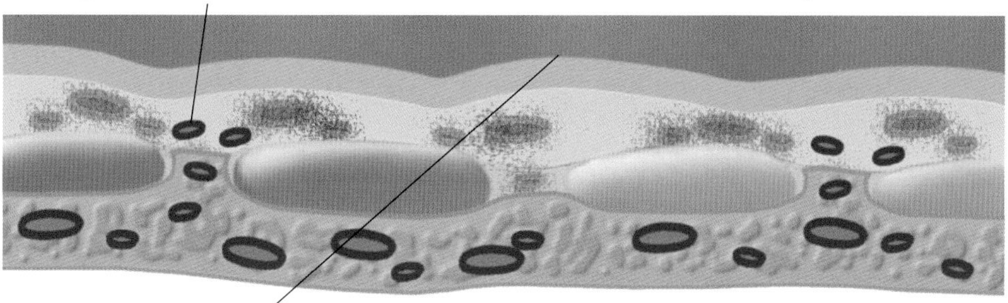

Ischemia of the mucosal lining (as seen during chronic rejection) will serve as a trigger for angiogenesis. Chronic rejection-induced ischemia will promote angiogenesis leading to graft endothelial repopulation.

"Art always develops due to new techniques and materials. Thanks to the evolution of 3D printing there is a whole world of new possibilities opening up for designing: possibilities of sculpting forms that were previously unthinkable."

NICK ERVINCK

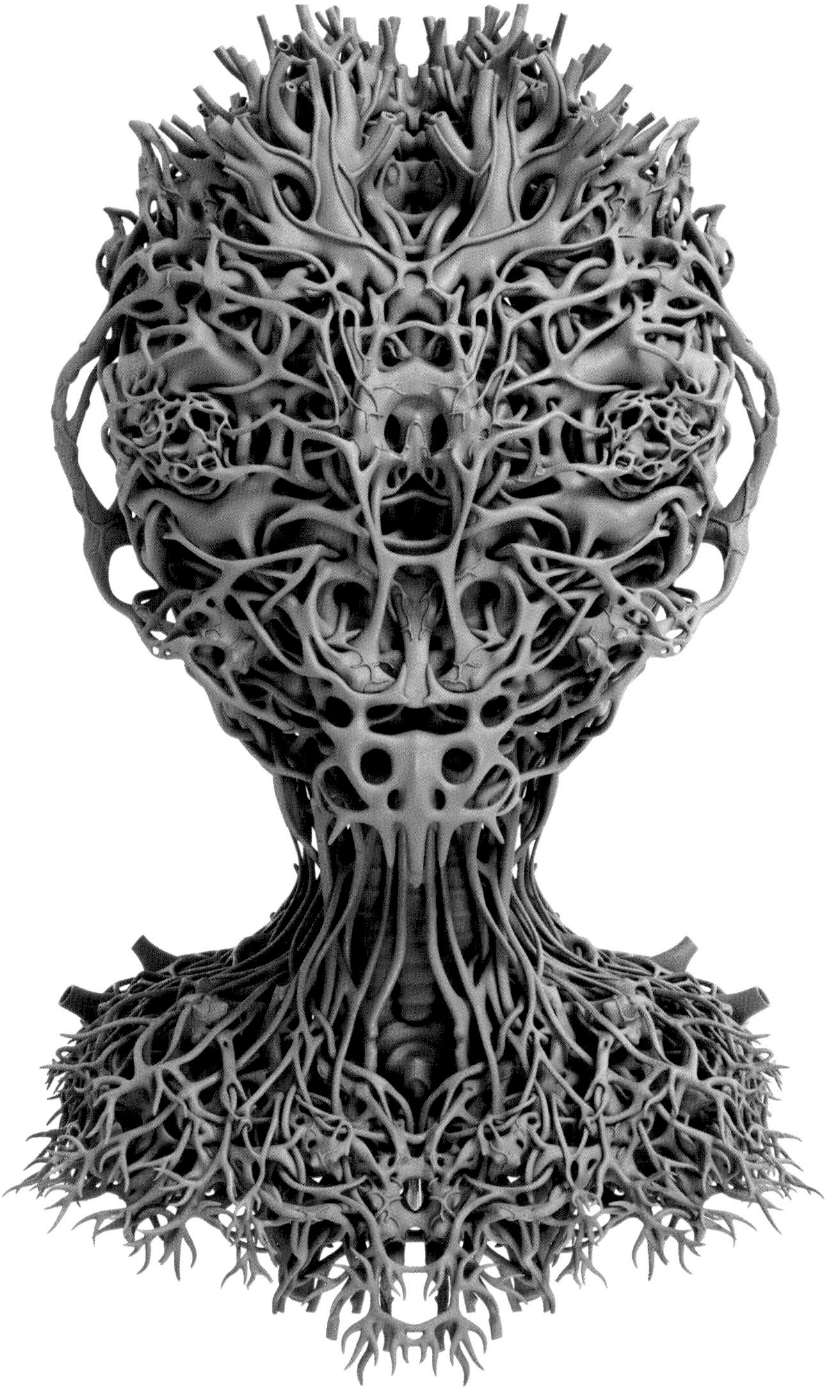

AGRIEBORZ, 2009-2011

3D PRINT – FRONTAL VIEW

53 × 34 × 33 CM

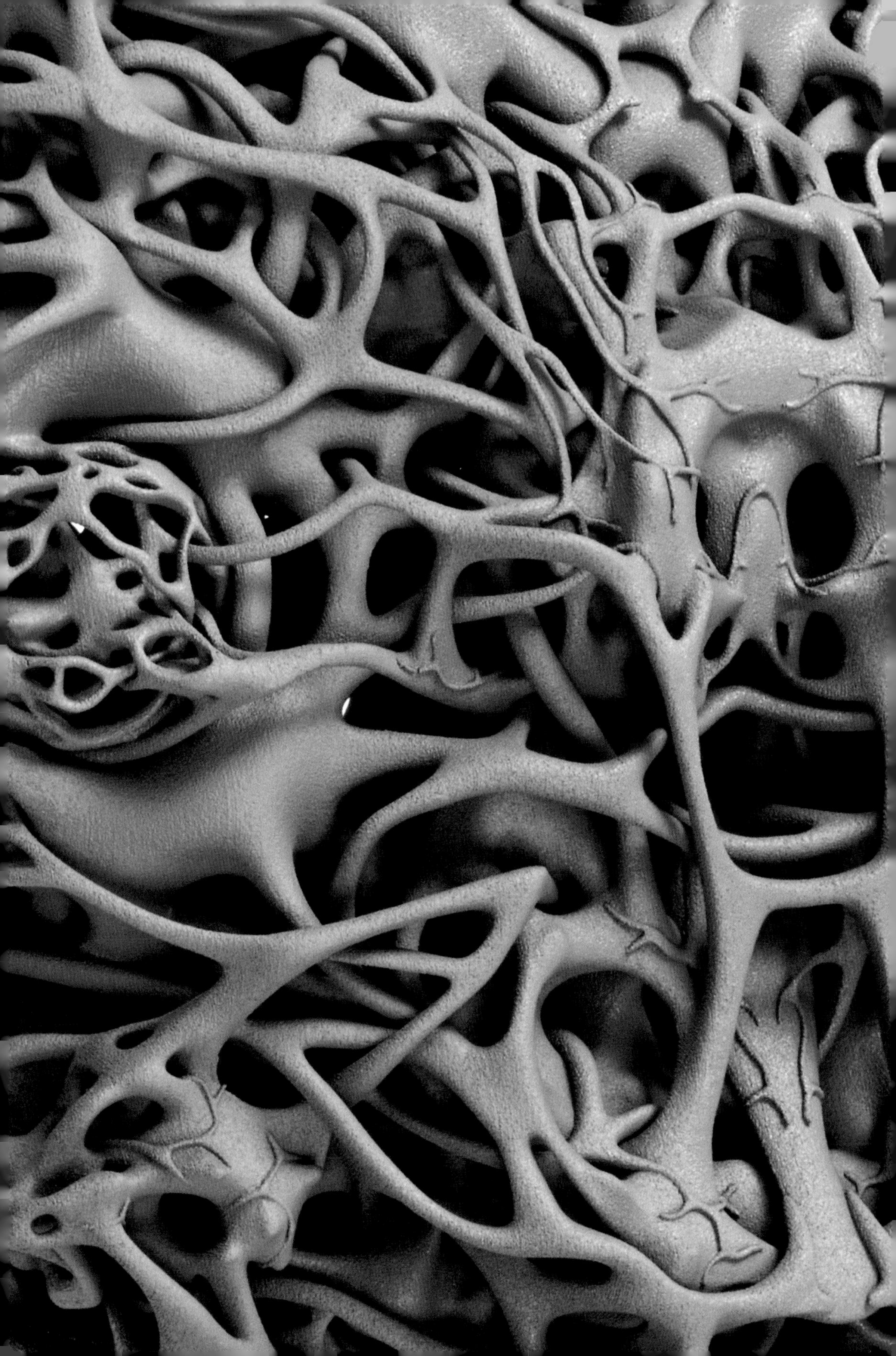

7. Tracheal allotransplantation – clinical aspects

Circumferential tracheal revascularization

Revascularization of the opened trachea (1) - (2) - (3)

Introduction of recipient buccal mucosa

Introduction of recipient skin graft

End-stage of tracheal revascularization

Role of intercartilaginous incisions

Tracheal chondrosarcoma – Preoperative CT scan

Tracheal chondrosarcoma – Heterotopic revascularization

Tracheal chondrosarcoma – Orthotopic transplantation

Tracheal chondrosarcoma – Postoperative CT scan

Withdrawal of immunosuppressive medication

Long-segment stenosis

Circumferential reconstruction (1) - (2)

Conclusion

We performed the first successful tracheal allotransplantation in 2008 (New Eng J Med, 2010). In our initial patient series, we explored the optimal position of the allotransplant in the forearm and obtained evidence for the importance of the intercartilaginous incisions in preserving full graft viability after the withdrawal of the immunosuppressive medication. This learning curve was published in 2012 (Am J Transpl). Our current experience includes seven transplants (6 long-segment stenosis and 1 tracheal chondrosarcoma).
In this chapter, our current approach is demonstrated.

Circumferential tracheal revascularization

FROM OUR FIRST PATIENT, WE LEARNED THAT CIRCUMFERENTIAL TRACHEAL WRAPPING IS NOT THE OPTIMAL APPROACH FOR TRACHEAL REVASCULARIZATION. CIRCUMFERENTIAL WRAPPING HAS TO BE AVOIDED BECAUSE OF THE TENDENCY OF THE MEMBRANOUS TRACHEA TO UNDERGO NECROSIS. NECROTIC TISSUE WITHIN THE TRACHEAL LUMEN, WHICH IS NOT AIRWAY EXPOSED, DO NOT PROVIDE THE OPTIMAL ENVIRONMENT FOR MUCOSAL REGENERATION.

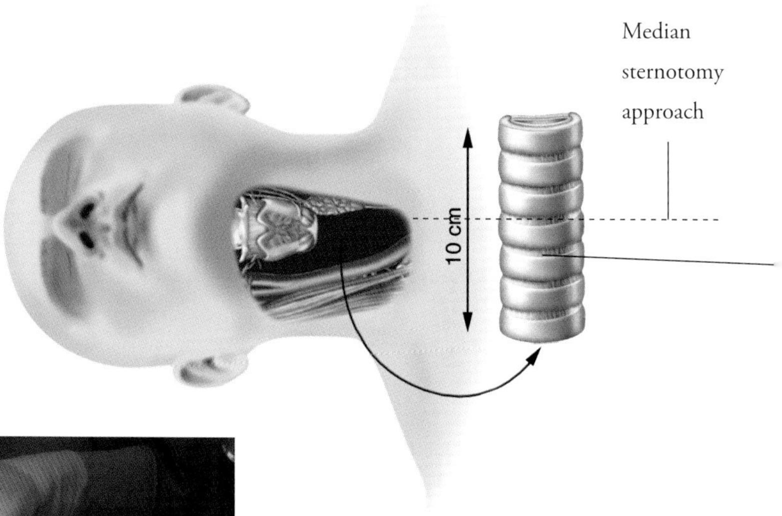
Median
sternotomy
approach
10 cm

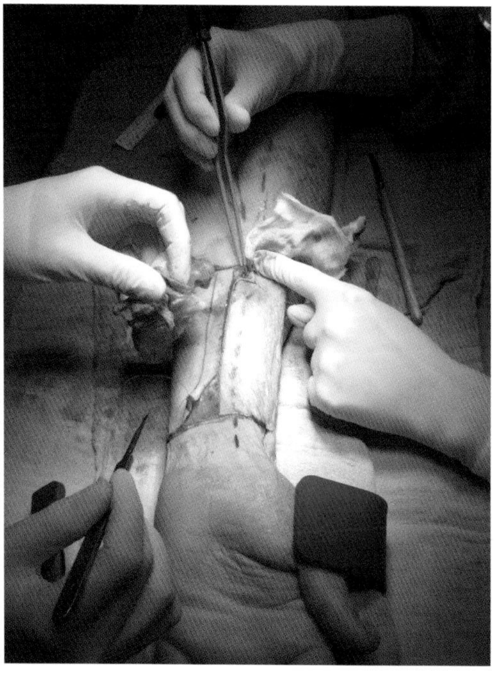

Skin flap incisions to approach the radial forearm fascia and subcutaneous tissue.

In our first patient, a tracheal segment was taken from a blood group-matched (heart beating) donor through a sternotomy approach during lung procurement. If necessary, the full tracheal length of the trachea can be taken and implanted in the forearm. In this patient, a tracheal allotransplant that was 10 cm in length was placed on the recipient forearm fascia within 12 hours.

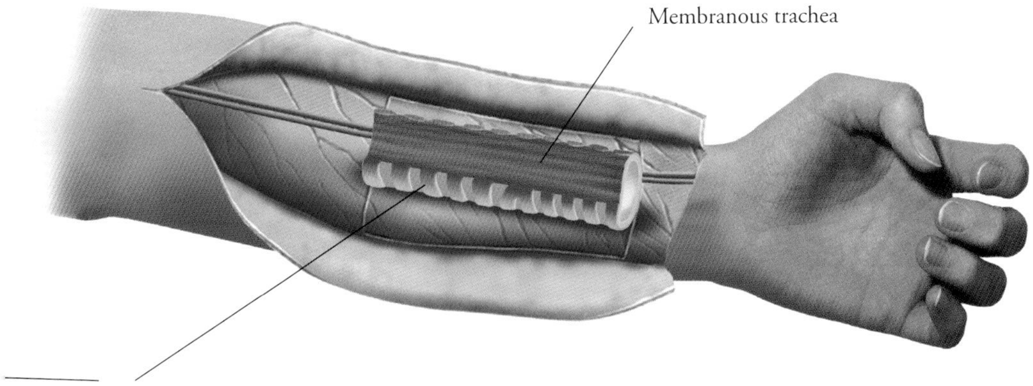
Membranous trachea
Tracheal allotransplant

FIRST PATIENT

In our first patient, the tracheal allotransplant was circumferentially wrapped with fascia. The membranous trachea underwent necrosis while the cartilaginous trachea displayed progressive revascularization. This was in contrast to the rabbit's trachea, which displayed a successful revascularization as a tube. The difference in revascularization can be explained by the different tracheal morphology (see page 101).

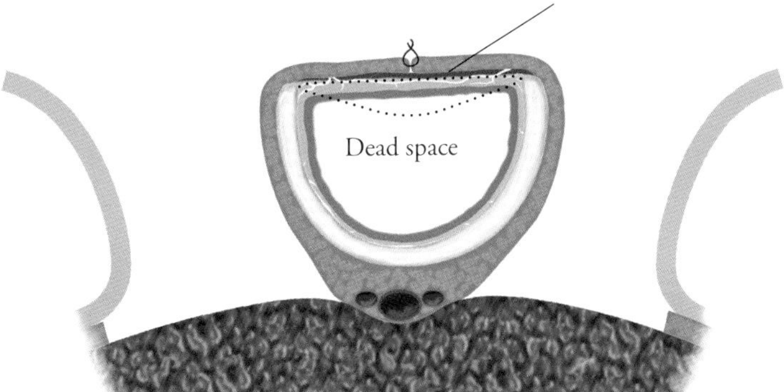
Necrosis of the membranous trachea
Dead space

Daily triple immunosuppression therapy:
- 6 mg tacrolimus
- 100 mg azathioprine
- 4 mg methylprednisolone

Revascularization of the opened trachea (1)

The intercartilaginous ligaments are partially incised at 1-cm intervals.

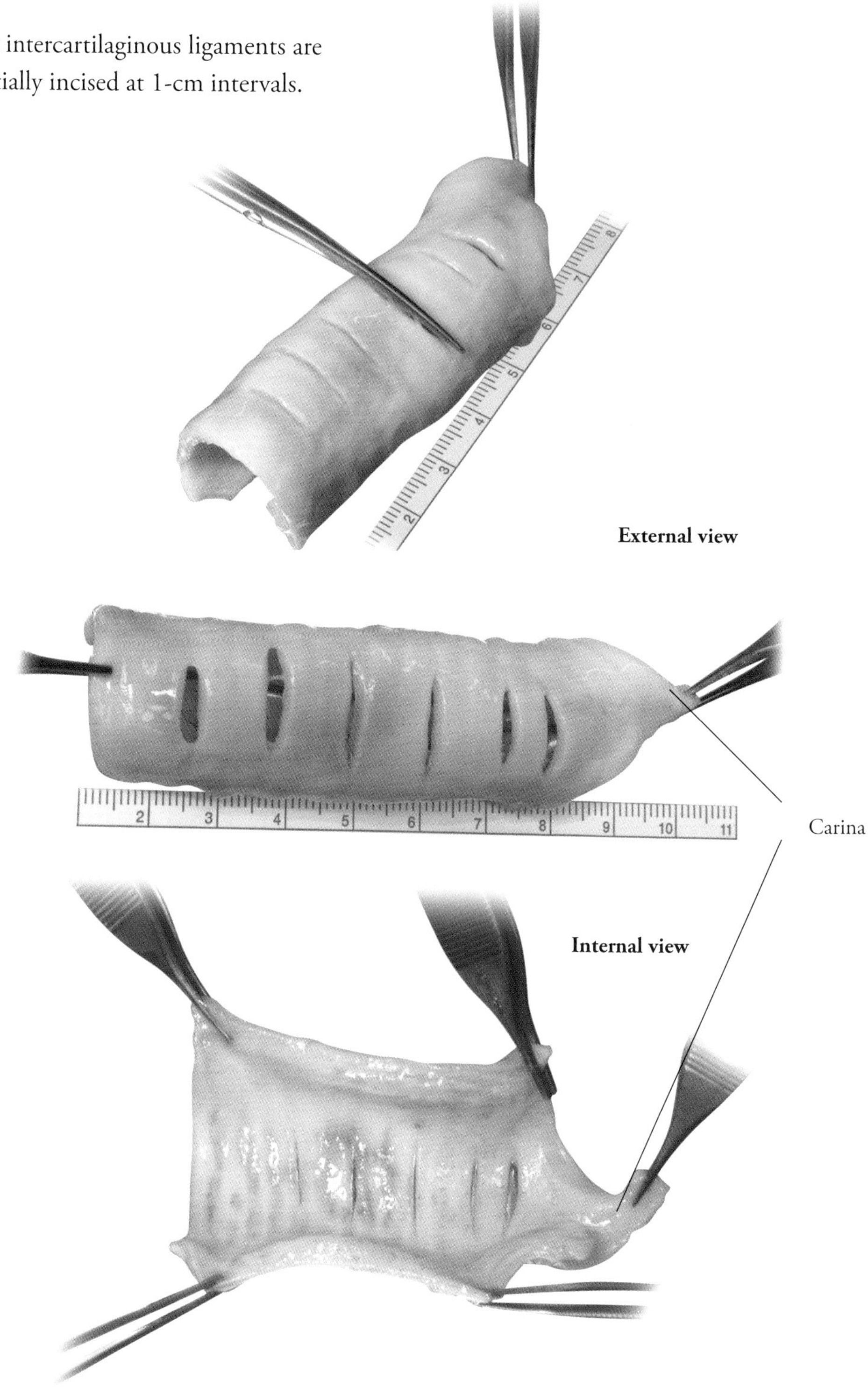
External view
Carina
Internal view

A BETTER OPTION FOR REVASCULARIZATION IS TO INCISE THE TRACHEA LONGITUDINALLY ALONG THE POSTERIOR MIDLINE. THIS ACTION EXPOSES THE TRACHEAL LUMEN AND MAKES IT ACCESSIBLE FOR CLEANING AND RINSING. THE INCISIONS OF THE INTERCARTILAGINOUS LIGAMENTS WILL FOSTER REVASCULARIZATION AND WILL ENABLE THE INGROWTH OF RECIPIENT VESSELS INTO THE SUBMUCOSAL SPACE OF THE TRANSPLANT.

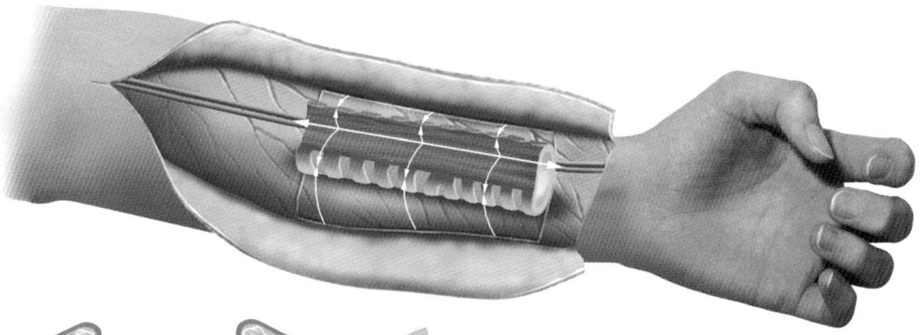

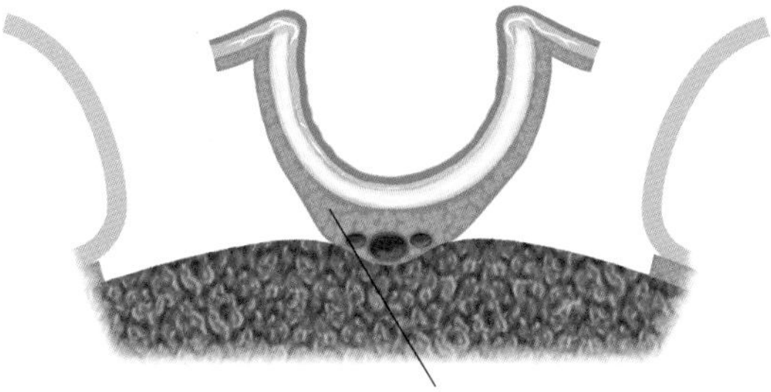

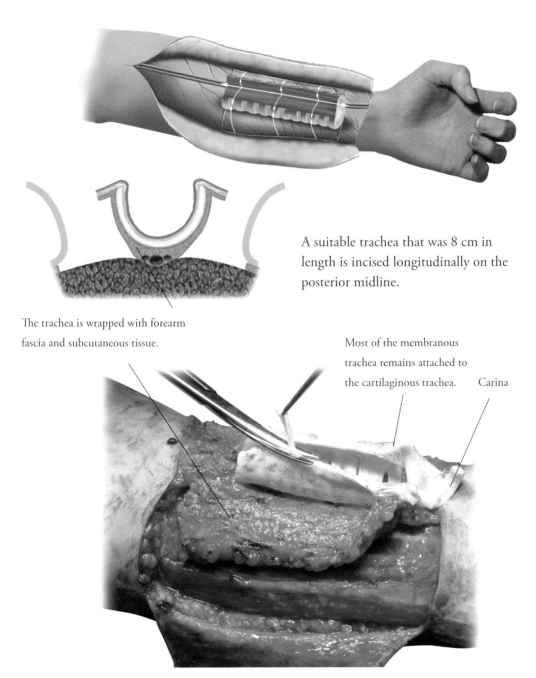

A suitable trachea that was 8 cm in length is incised longitudinally on the posterior midline.

The trachea is wrapped with forearm fascia and subcutaneous tissue.

Most of the membranous trachea remains attached to the cartilaginous trachea.

Carina

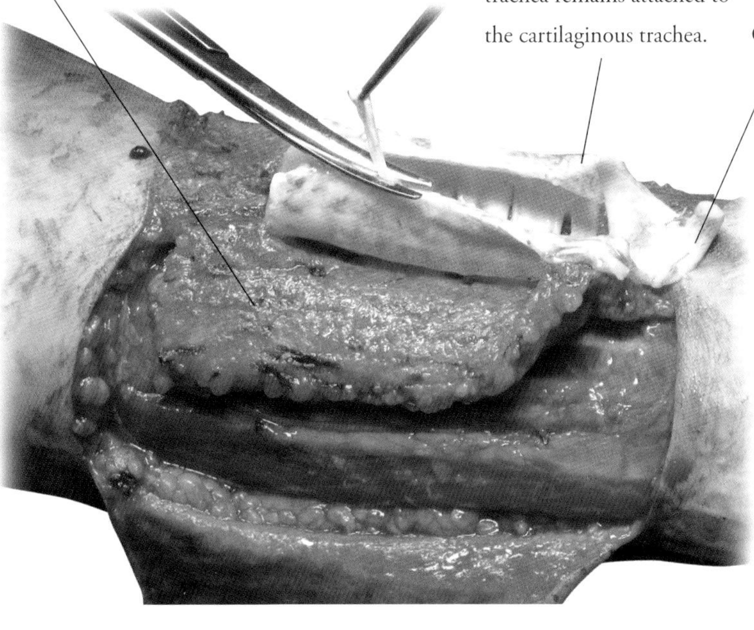

Revascularization of the opened trachea (2)

THE APPEARANCE OF THE FOREARM IMMEDIATELY AFTER INSETTING OF THE TRACHEAL ALLOTRANSPLANT.

Intercartilaginous ligaments will fasten the revascularization process and the ingrowth of recipient blood vessels from the fascia into the submucosal space of the transplant.

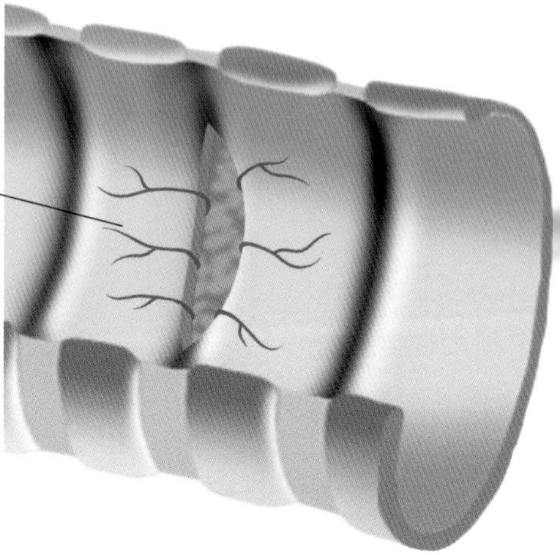

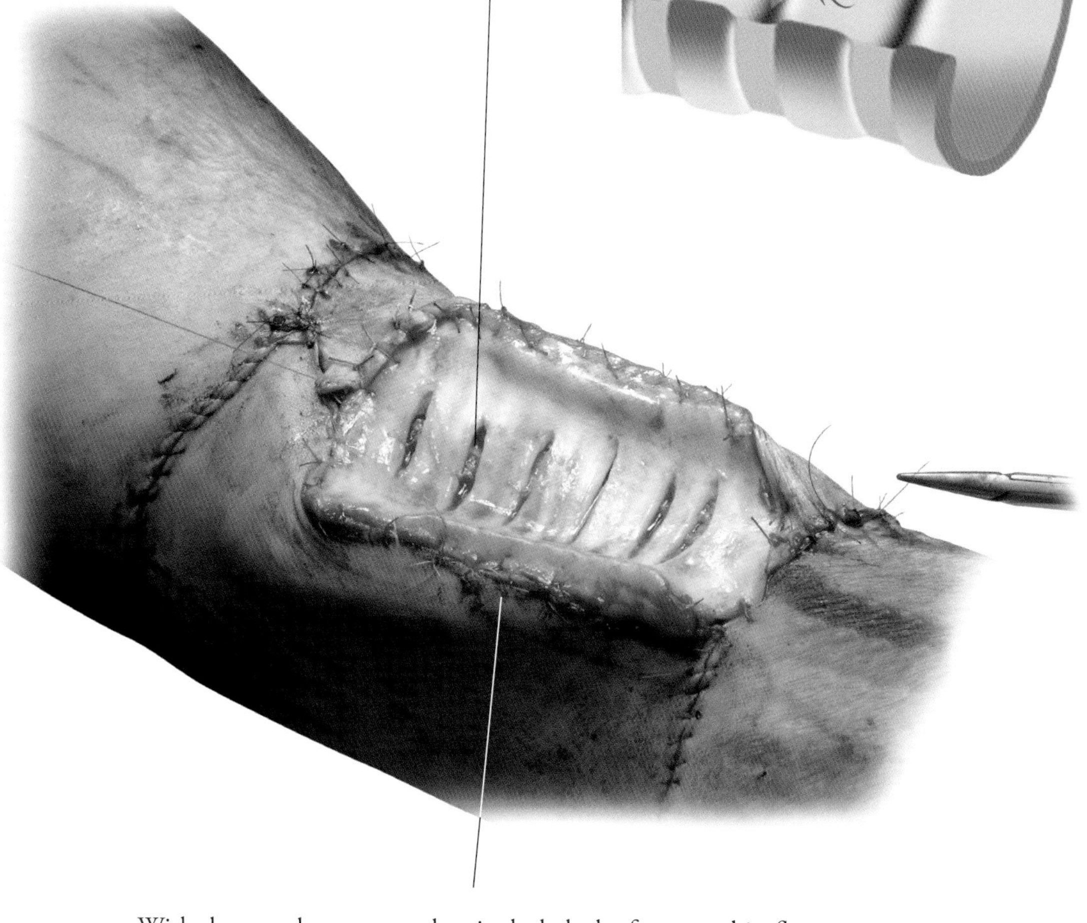

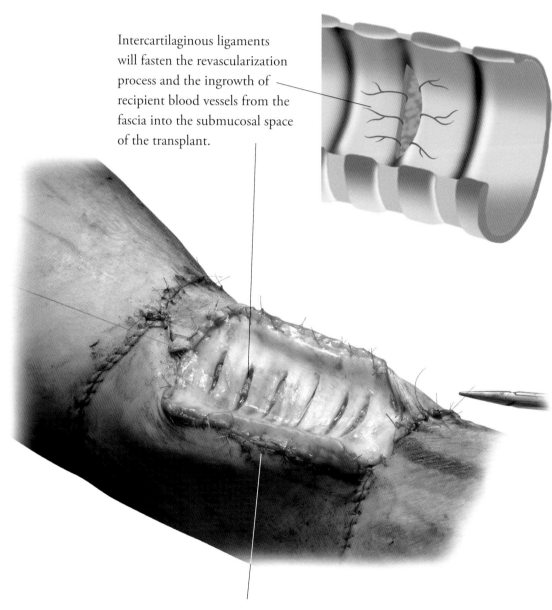

With the membranous trachea included, the forearm skin flap can be sutured without tension to the tracheal allotransplant.

Detail of membranous trachea

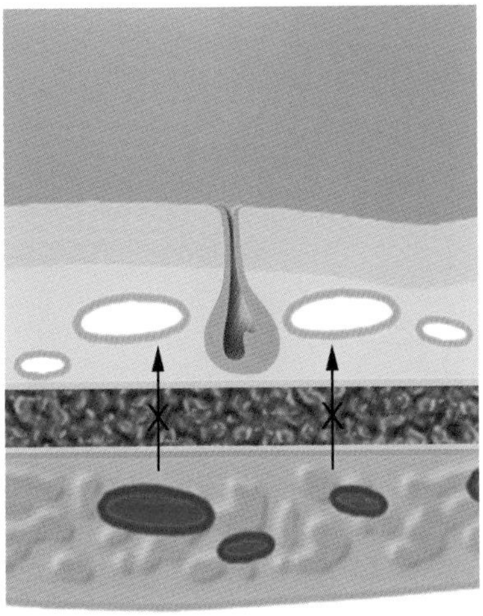

The trachealis muscle forms an obstacle for the revascularization of the membranous trachea.

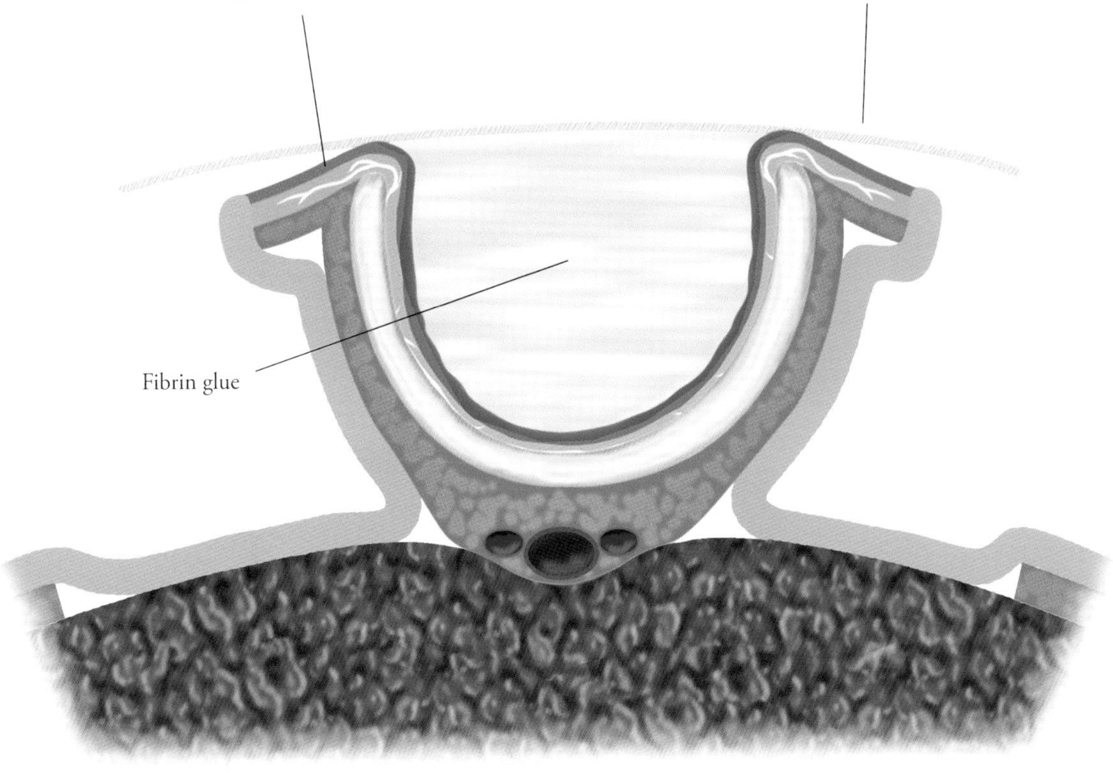
The membranous trachea remains attached to the cartilaginous trachea
Gore-Tex® sheet
Fibrin glue

After forearm implantation, the luminal site of the transplant is protected by the application of fibrin glue. A Gore-Tex® sheet covers the transplant.

Revascularization of the opened trachea (3)

PROGRESSIVE REVASCULARIZATION AND MUCOSAL REGENERATION WILL OCCUR OVER A 2-MONTH PERIOD.

SITUATION AFTER 2 WEEKS

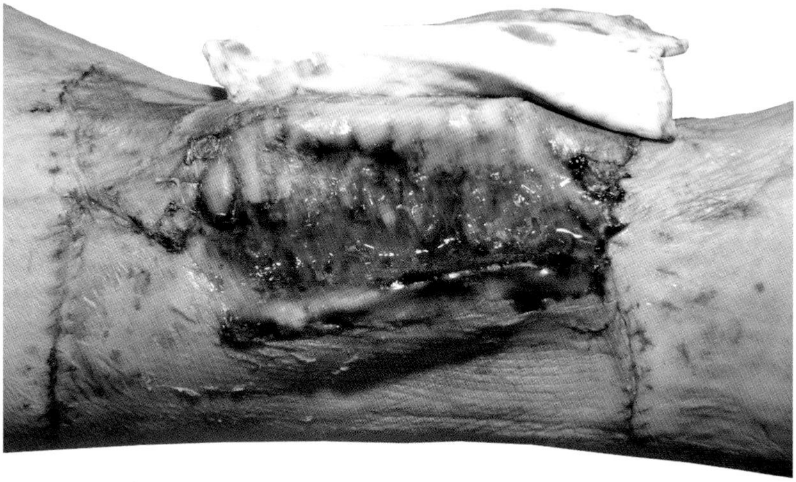

The internal site of the transplant is evaluated every week.

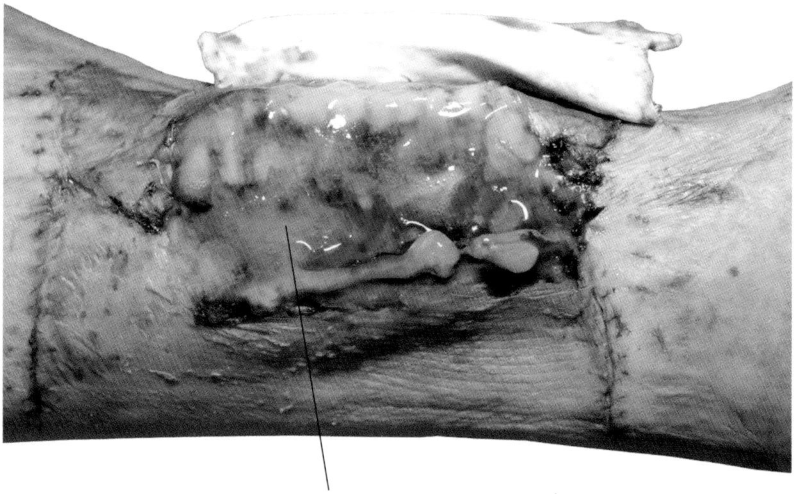

PROTECTION OF THE MUCOSAL LINING

During the first weeks, the mucosal lining is protected from drying out with fibrin glue. After 3 weeks, the patient is asked to rinse the transplant with saline three times per day. It is important to keep the mucosal lining moist.

SITUATION AFTER 5 WEEKS

A Gore-Tex® soft tissue patch protects the tracheal transplant

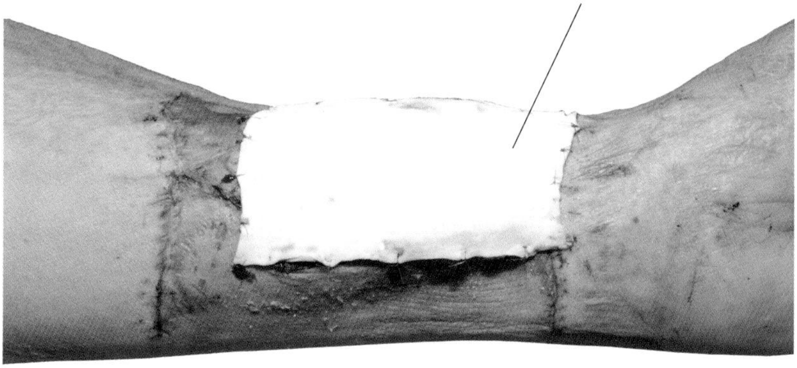

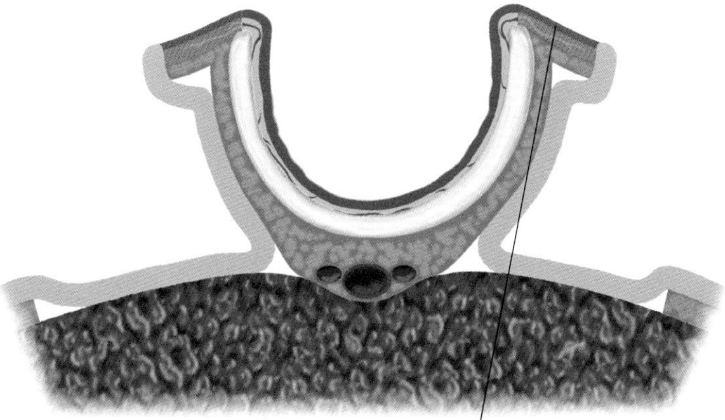

The membranous trachea has a tendency to undergo necrosis.

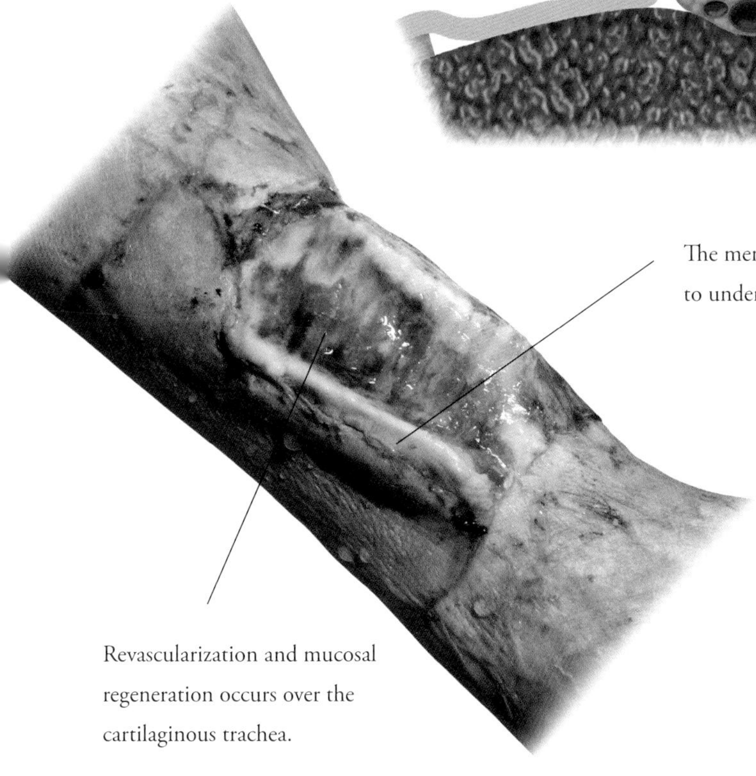

Revascularization and mucosal regeneration occurs over the cartilaginous trachea.

Introduction of recipient buccal mucosa

FULL REVASCULARIZATION OF THE CARTILAGINOUS TRACHEA WILL BE OBTAINED TWO MONTHS AFTER IMPLANTATION IN THE FOREARM. AT THAT TIME, RECIPIENT BUCCAL MUCOSA CAN BE INTRODUCED INTO THE MIDPORTION OF THE ALLOTRANSPLANT.

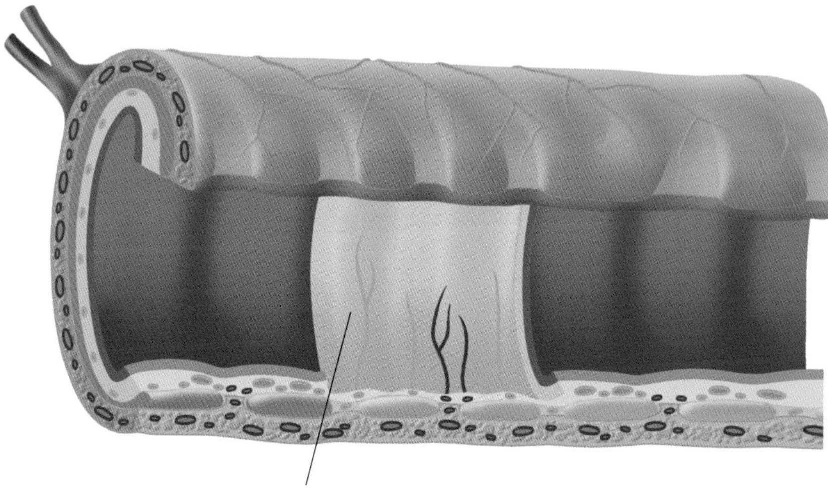

A full-thickness mucosal defect is created in the central part of the transplant.

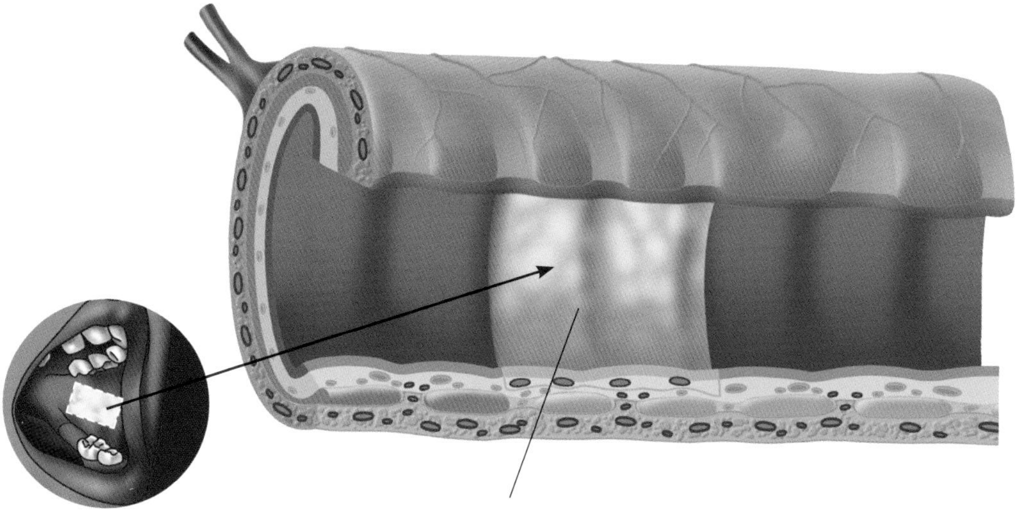

The midportion is grafted with a full-thickness mucosa graft from the recipient's buccal area.

Outlining of mucosal defect in the central part of the transplant.

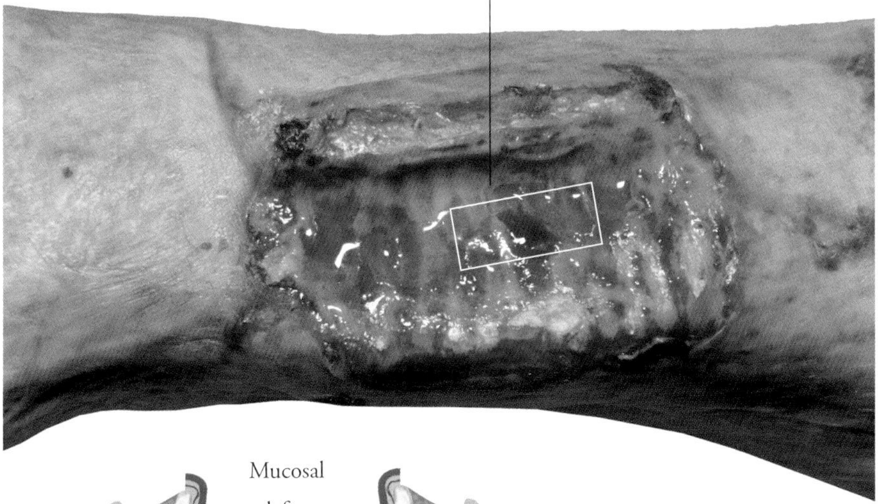

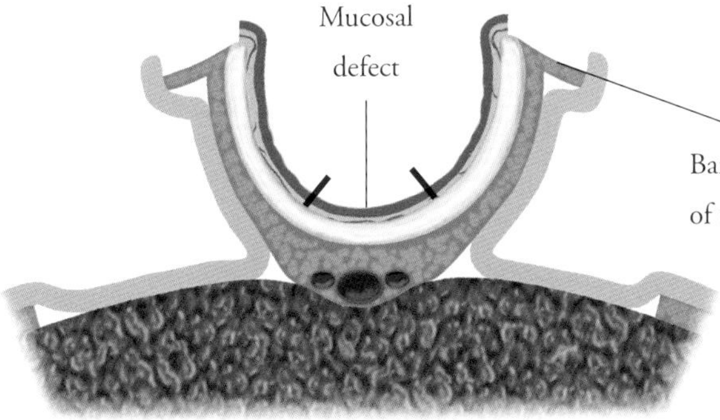
Mucosal
defect

Bare fascia after necrosis
of the membranous trachea.

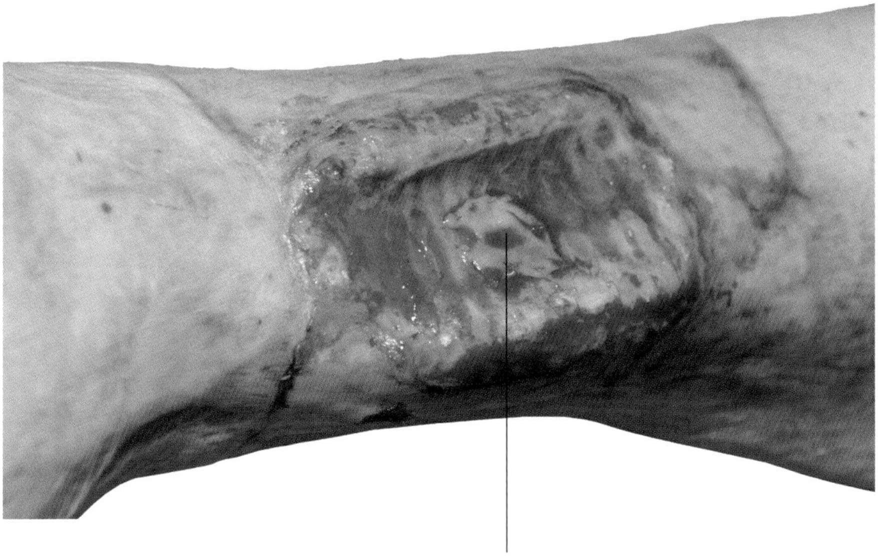

Full-thickness buccal mucosa graft. Insetting is performed with interrupted Vicryl 5.0 sutures.

Introduction of recipient skin graft

IT IS ADVISABLE TO INTRODUCE SOME ADDITIONAL EPITHELIAL LINING FROM A SKIN GRAFT. DURING THE SAME OPERATIVE SESSION AS THE BUCCAL MUCOSAL GRAFTING, A MESHED, SPLIT-THICKNESS SKIN GRAFT IS DRAPED OVER THE INTERNAL SITE OF THE TRACHEAL ALLOTRANSPLANT. THE ADDITIONAL RECIPIENT EPITHELIAL CELLS MAY HELP IN THE HEALING PROCESS OF THE TRACHEAL TRANSPLANT'S LINING AFTER THE WITHDRAWAL OF IMMUNOSUPPRESSIVE DRUGS.

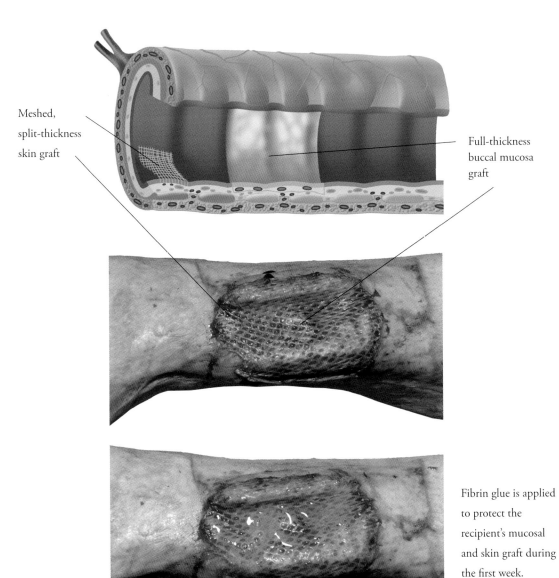

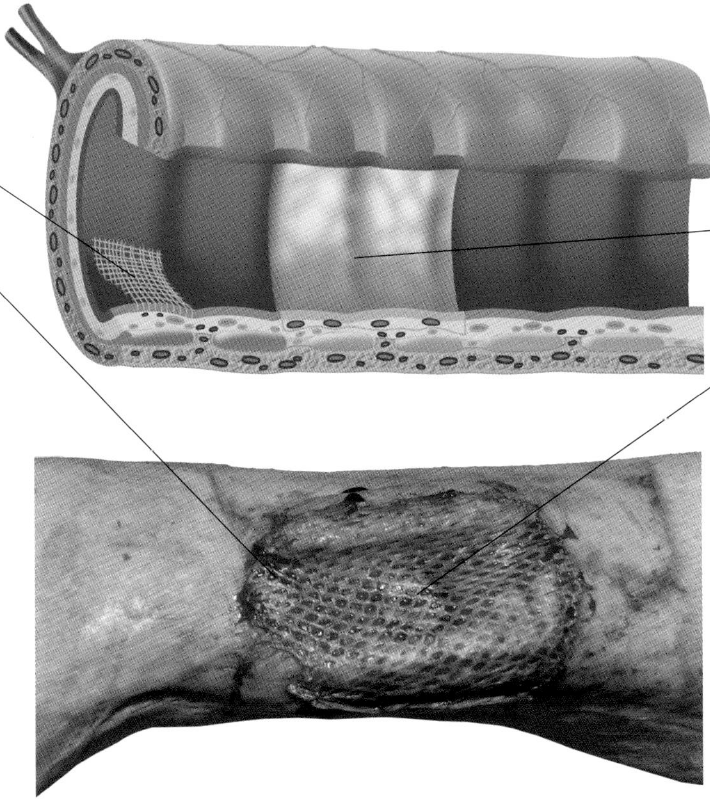
Meshed, split-thickness skin graft
Full-thickness buccal mucosa graft

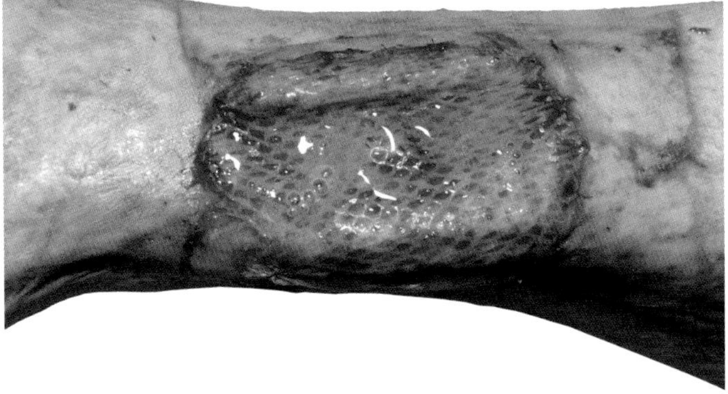

Fibrin glue is applied to protect the recipient's mucosal and skin graft during the first week.

SPLIT-THICKNESS SKIN GRAFT

The graft will survive at the sites with incomplete donor epithelial regeneration. The graft will underdo necrosis at the sites already covered with donor or recipient epithelium.

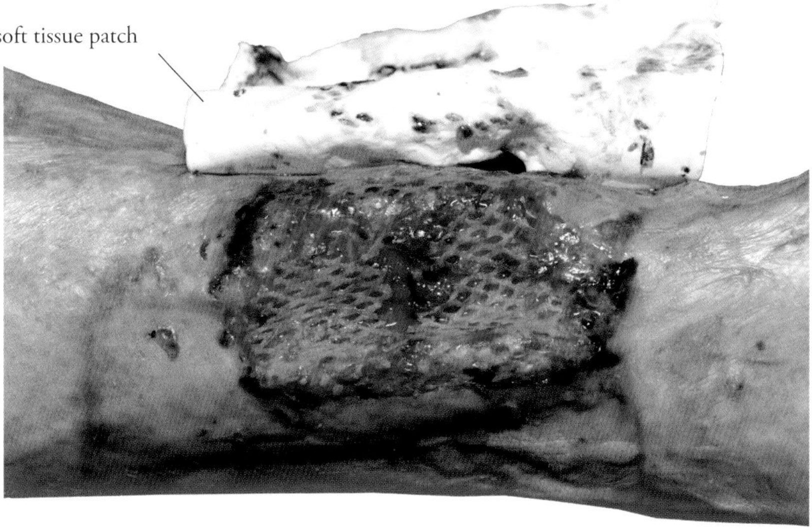
Gore-Tex® soft tissue patch

1 week after the recipient's epithelium grafting

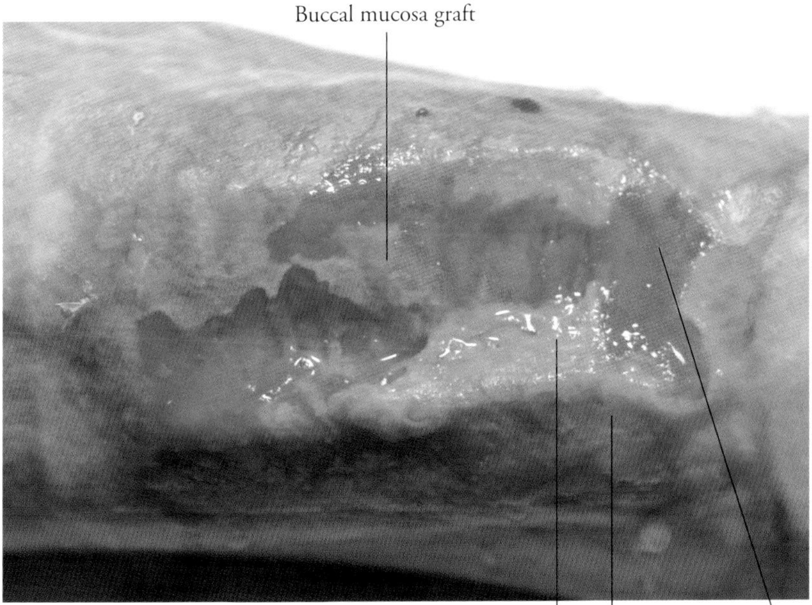
Buccal mucosa graft
Split-thickness skin graft
Respiratory epithelium (donor)

2 weeks after the recipient's epithelium grafting

The mucosal lining has to remain wet by daily (3x) rinsing with saline.

End-stage of tracheal revascularization

IMMUNOSUPPRESSION

The tracheal transplant appears as a chimera that consists of different donor and recipient tissues.

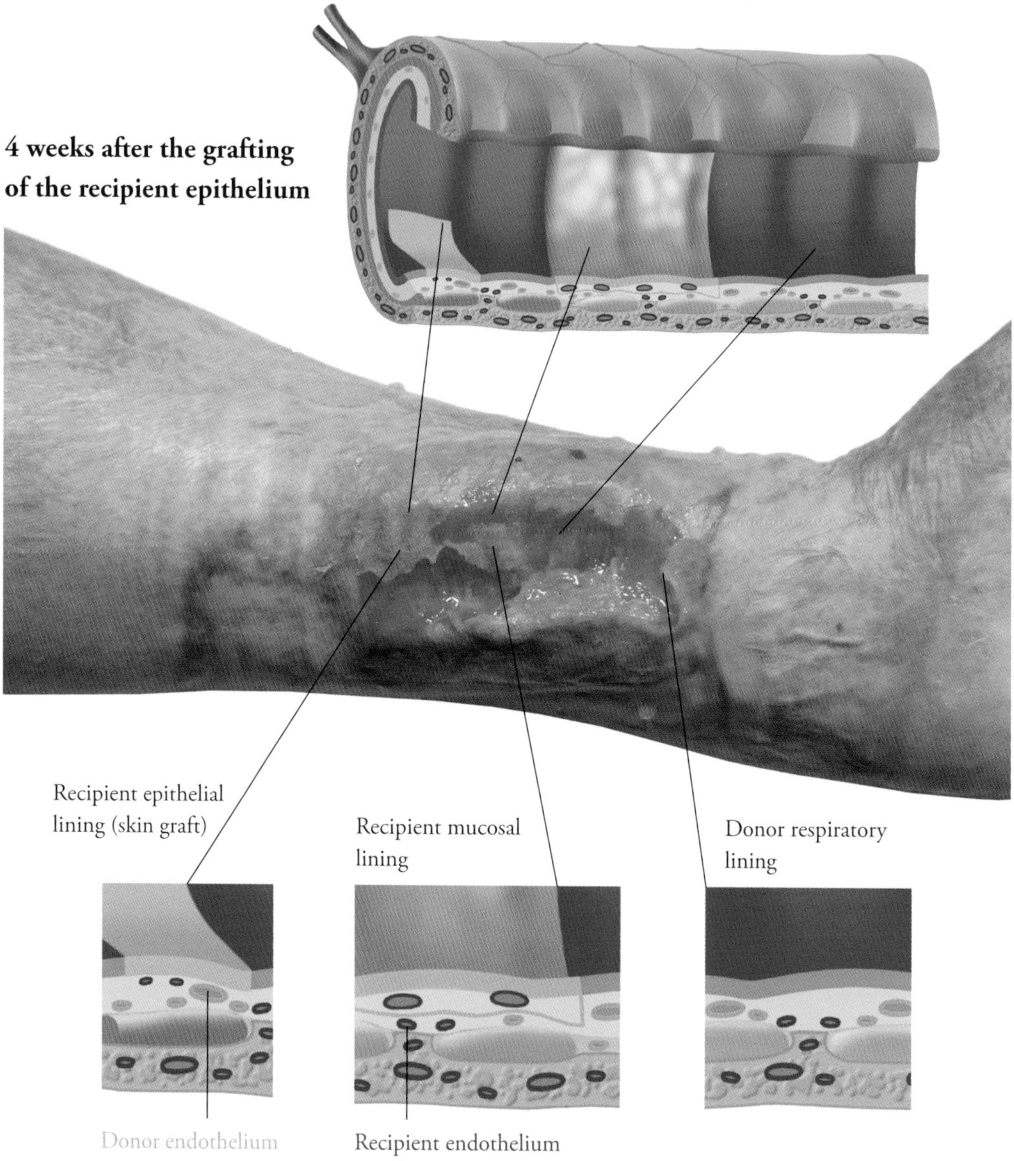
4 weeks after the grafting of the recipient epithelium
Recipient epithelial lining (skin graft)
Recipient mucosal lining
Donor respiratory lining
Donor endothelium
Recipient endothelium

THE REVASCULARIZED ALLOTRANSPLANT CONSISTS OF DIFFERENT RECIPIENT AND DONOR TISSUES. THE DONOR'S EPITHELIAL LINING AND ENDOTHELIUM WILL DISAPPEAR AFTER THE WITHDRAWAL (STARTING ONE YEAR AFTER ORTHOTOPIC TRANSPLANTATION) OF IMMUNOSUPPRESSIVE MEDICATION. THESE AREAS NEED TO BECOME REPOPULATED BY RECIPIENT VESSELS AND RECIPIENT EPITHELIUM. THE REPOPULATION PROCESS NEEDS TO BE GRADUAL WITH NO OR MINIMAL SECONDARY HEALING AND MINIMAL LOSS OF THE AIRWAY LUMEN.

AFTER THE WITHDRAWAL OF IMMUNOSUPPRESSION
(one year after orthotopic transplantation)

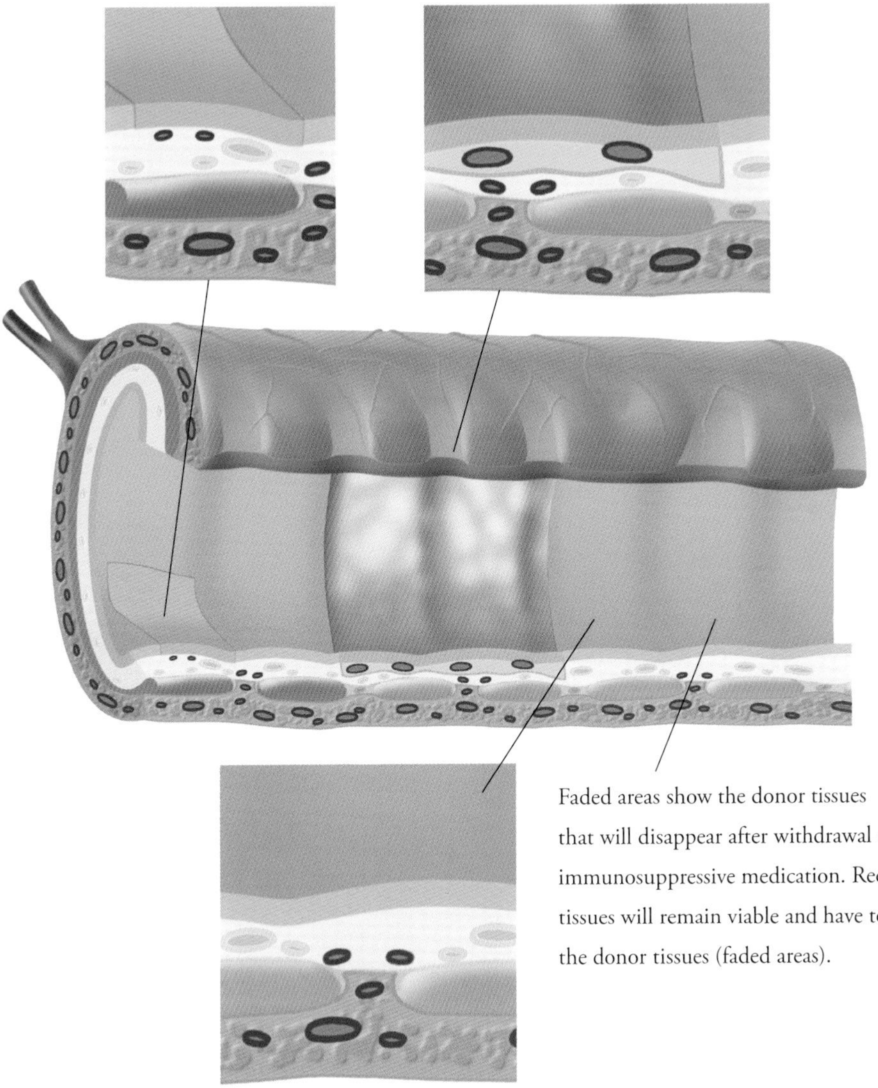

Faded areas show the donor tissues that will disappear after withdrawal of immunosuppressive medication. Recipient tissues will remain viable and have to replace the donor tissues (faded areas).

Role of intercartilaginous incisions

ADDITIONAL MEASURES WILL BE NECESSARY TO OPTIMIZE TRACHEAL TRANSPLANT SURVIVAL AFTER THE WITHDRAWAL OF IMMUNOSUPRESSIVE DRUGS. MOST IMPORTANT WILL BE THE GROWTH OF RECIPIENT BLOOD VESSELS IN THE SUBMUCOSAL SPACE OF THE GRAFT. THIS CAN BE GUARANTEED BY MAKING PARTIAL INCISIONS THROUGH THE INTERCARTILAGINOUS LIGAMENTS.

WITHOUT INCISIONS AFTER WITHDRAWAL OF IMMUNOSUPPRESSIVE MEDICATION

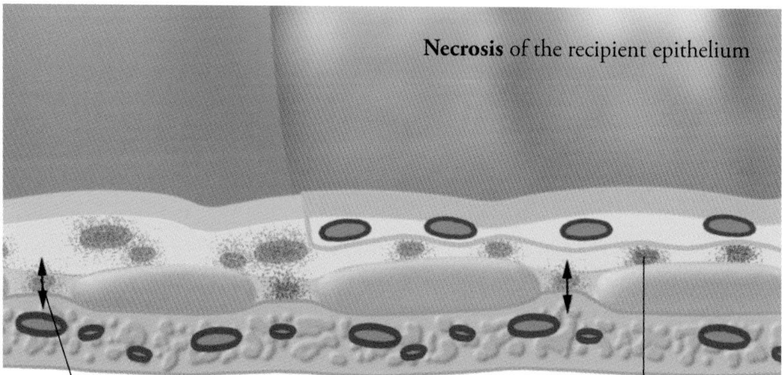
Necrosis of the recipient epithelium

Thrombosis of donor capillaries

Incisions at the intercartilaginous ligaments at the time of forearm implantation will allow for the ingrowth of recipient blood vessels.

Necrosis of the buccal mucosa graft after the cessation of immunosuppression should be avoided after the intercartilaginous incisions are made.

Ingrowth of recipient vessels

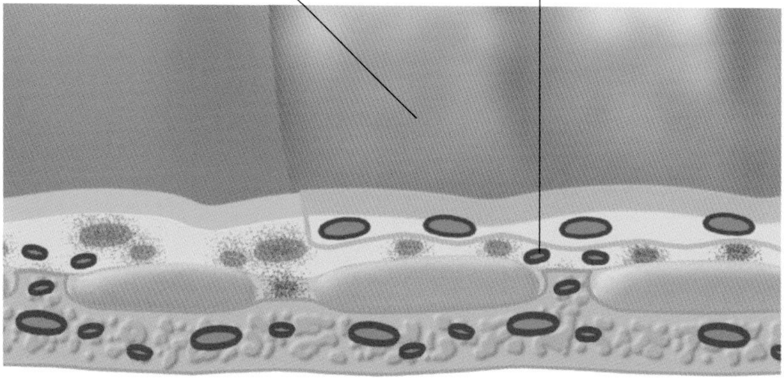

WITH INCISIONS AFTER WITHDRAWAL OF IMMUNOSUPPRESSIVE MEDICATION

THESE INCISIONS WILL DISRUPT THE BARRIER FOR THE ANGIOGENETIC OUTGROWTH OF RECIPIENT VESSELS TOWARDS THE SUBMUCOSAL SPACE OF THE TRANSPLANT. THE RECIPIENT VESSELS WILL ENABLE THE SURVIVAL OF THE RECIPIENT'S EPITHELIAL LINING IN THE MIDPORTION OF THE TRANSPLANT.

Intercartilaginous incisions and survival of the mucosal lining in the midportion of the allotranplant after the withdrawal of immunosuppressive medication

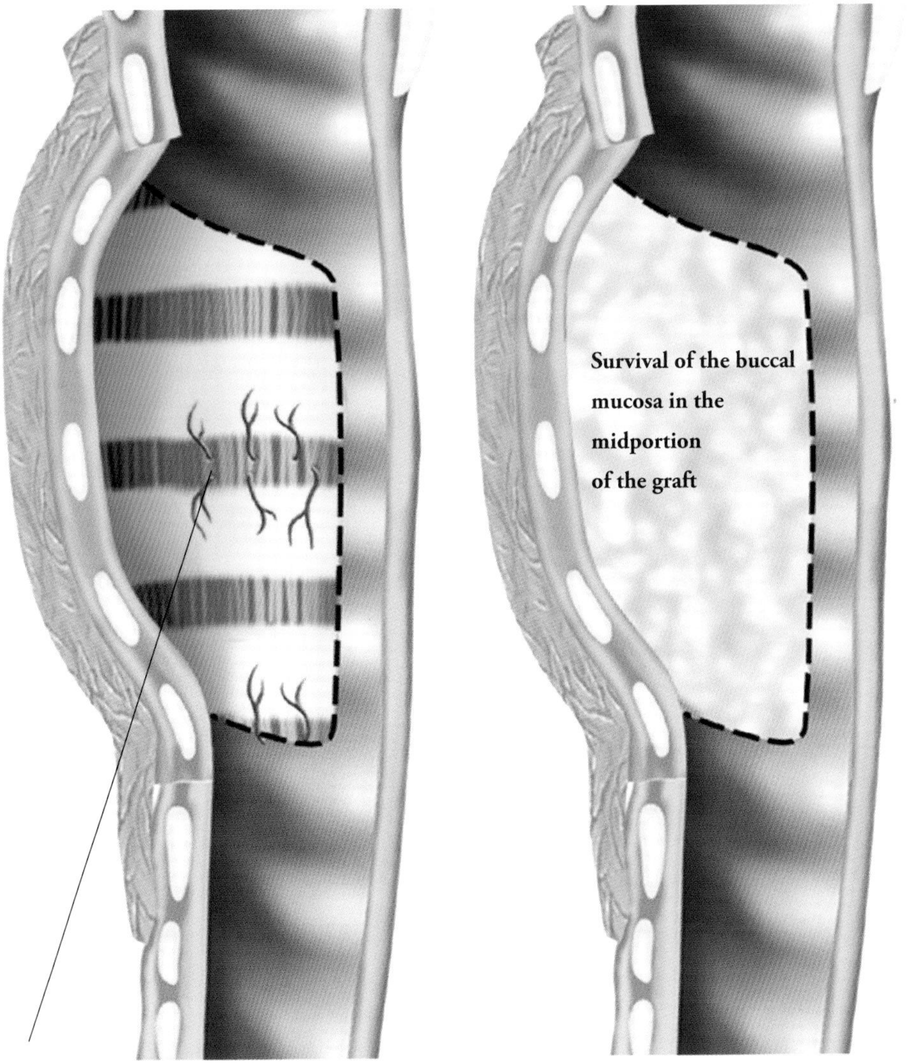
Survival of the buccal
mucosa in the
midportion
of the graft

Ingrowth of the recipient blood vessels at the site of an intercartilaginous ligament incision

Tracheal chondrosarcoma – Preoperative CT scan

TRACHEAL ALLOTRANSPLANTATION WAS USED IN THE TREATMENT OF A PATIENT WITH AN EXTENDED LARYNGOTRACHEAL CHONDROSARCOMA. THE PATIENT INVOLVED WAS A 63-YEAR-OLD MAN.

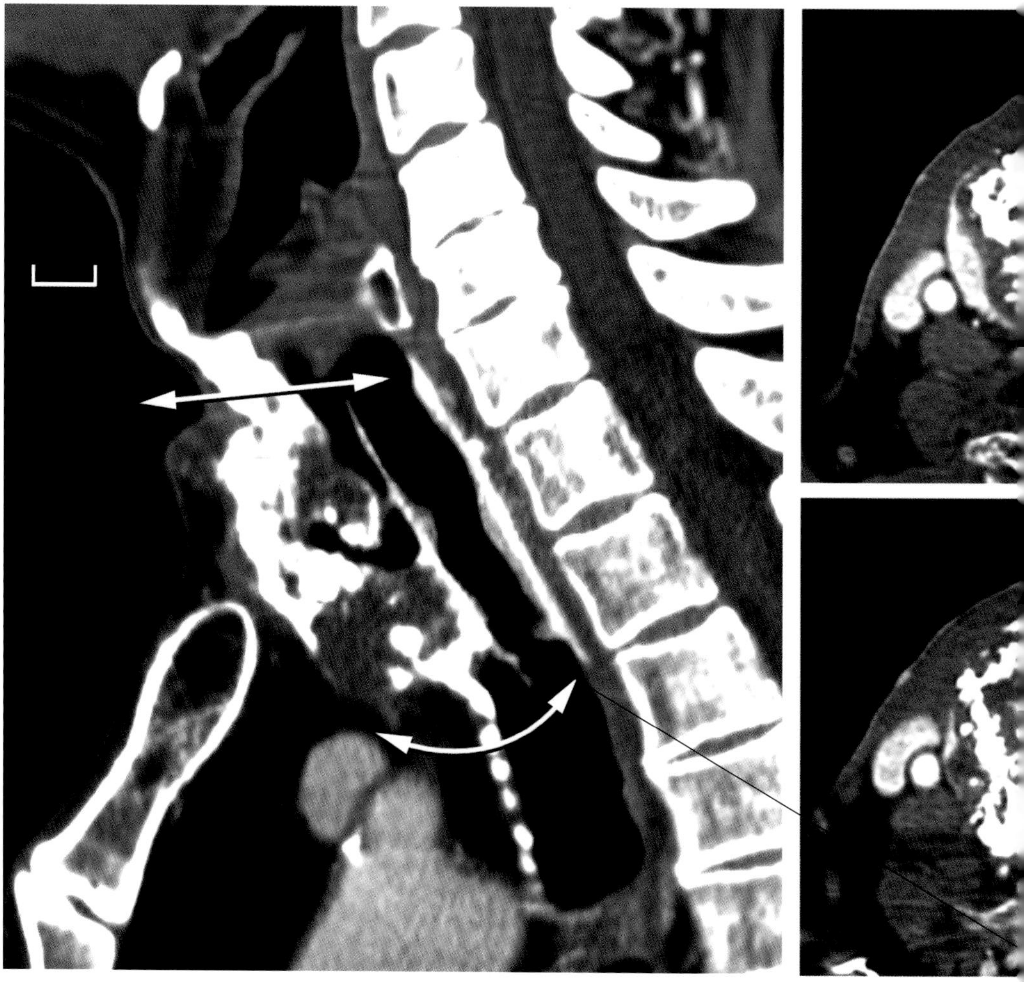

Tumor involvement visible on the sagittal, axial, and coronal CT scan images. The airway lumen is bridged by a silicone stent. The degree of resection is indicated with white, two-headed arrows. The lengths of the tracheal resection were 9 cm (right) and 6 cm (left) (scale = 1 cm).

THE TUMOR DEVELOPED OVER A PERIOD OF MORE THAN 10 YEARS. HIS AIRWAY COULD BE PRESERVED BY THE PLACEMENT OF A SILICONE STENT. DUE TO THE STAGNATION OF SECRETIONS, HE REQUIRED PERIODICAL BRONCHOSCOPIC CLEANING OF THE STENT. SINCE THE LAST TIME, HE HAD DEVELOPED SEVERAL ACUTE EPISODES OF STENT BLOCKAGES, WHICH MADE DEFINITIVE TREATMENT NECESSARY. BEFORE TUMOR RESECTION, A SUITABLE (BLOOD GROUP MATCHED) ALLOTRANSPLANT WAS SOUGHT.

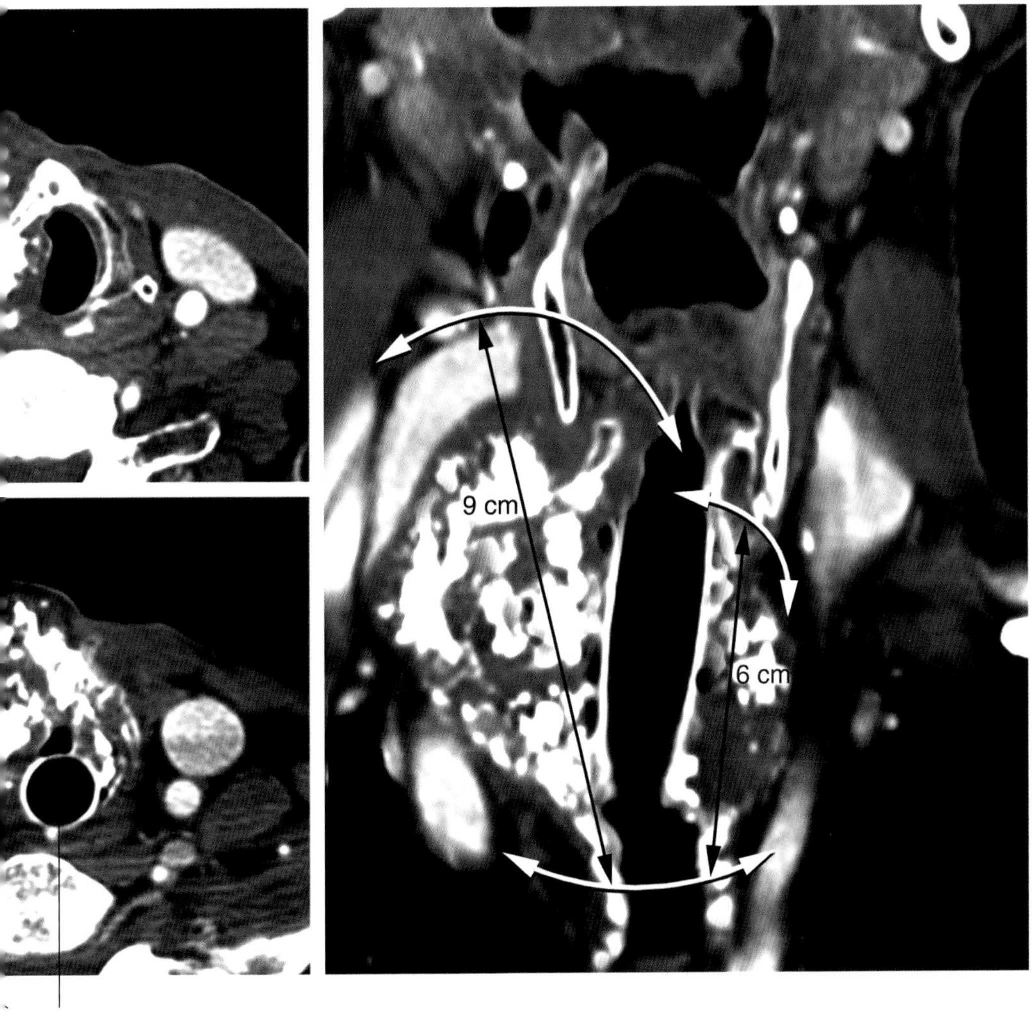
9 cm
6 cm
Tracheal stent

> "The potential for tumor progression while under immunosuppression for a low-grade malignancy was considered to be low and was confirmed by CT scan at the time of orthotopic transplantation, which demonstrated a nearly unchanged tumor bulk".

Tracheal chondrosarcoma – Heterotopic revascularization

THE ALLOGRAFT WAS REVASCULARIZED AND REMUCOSALIZED AT ITS MIDPORTION. AFTER 3 MONTHS, THE TUMOR COULD BE RESECTED AND THE TRACHEAL ALLOTRANSPLANT WAS USED TO REPAIR THE LARYNGOTRACHEAL DEFECT.

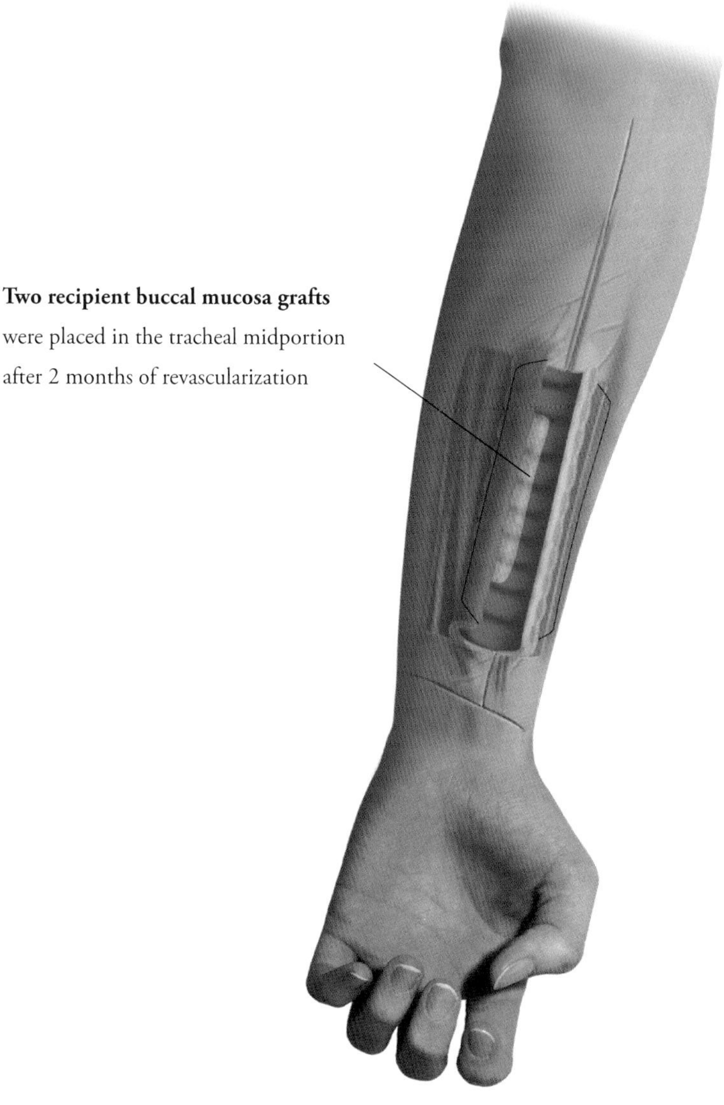
Two recipient buccal mucosa grafts
were placed in the tracheal midportion
after 2 months of revascularization

The allograft was transplanted into the laryngeal defect after 3 months.

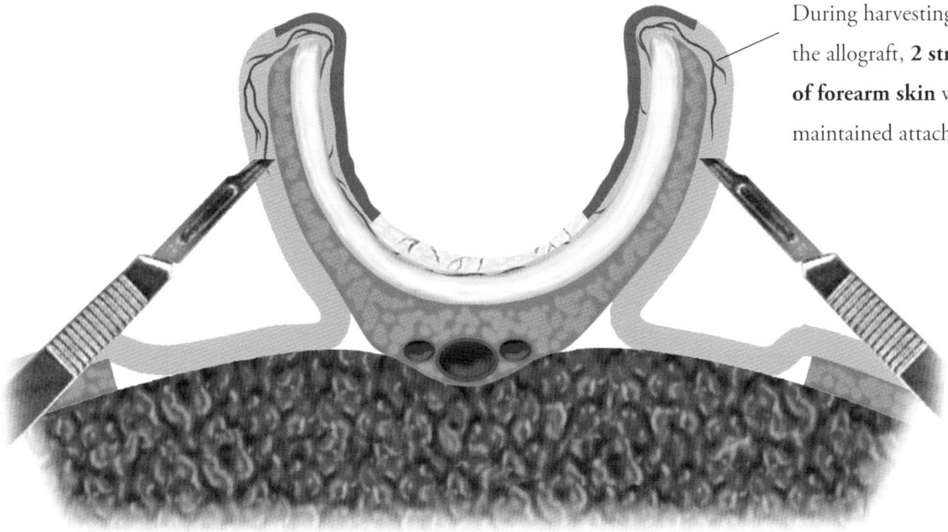

During harvesting of the allograft, **2 strips of forearm skin** were maintained attached.

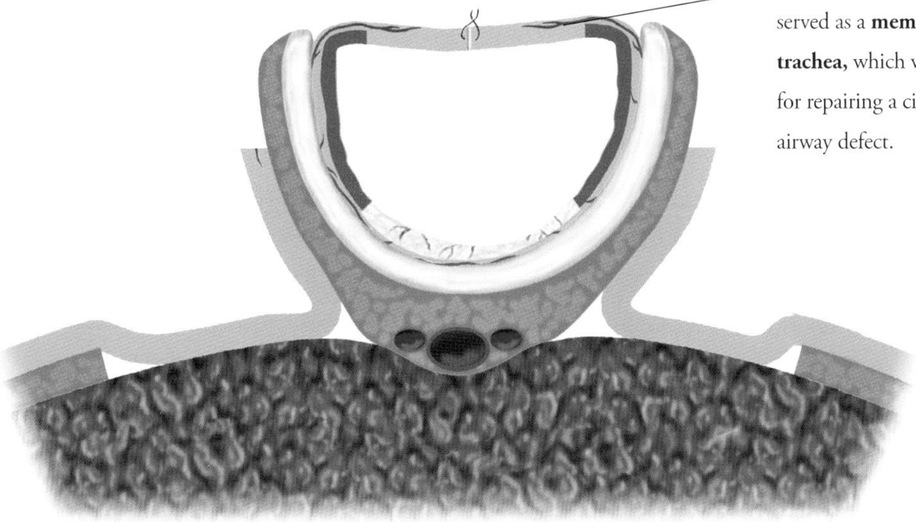

The strips of forearm skin served as a **membranous trachea,** which were useful for repairing a circumferential airway defect.

Tracheal chondrosarcoma – Orthotopic transplantation

AFTER 3 MONTHS OF ALLOTRANSPLANT REVASCULARIZATION, THE TUMOR WAS RESECTED THROUGH AN ANTERIOR CERVICAL INCISION WITH A STERNOTOMY EXTENSION.

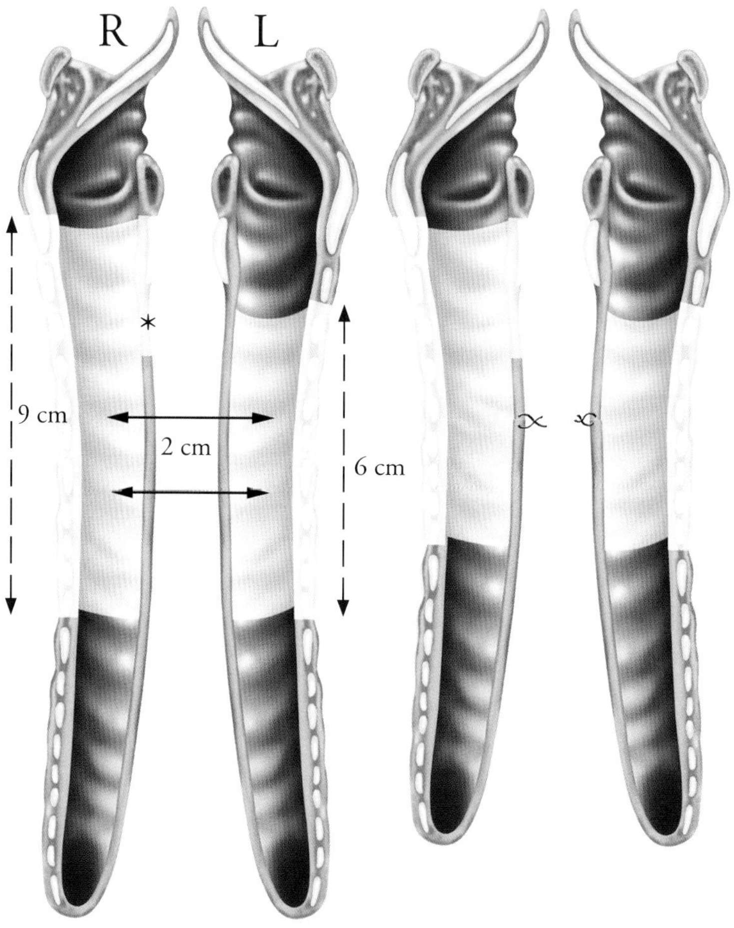
R
L
*
9 cm
2 cm
6 cm

LARYNGOTRACHEAL DEFECT

The length of the laryngotracheal defect on the right measured 9 cm; the tracheal defect on the left side measured 6 cm. Most of the membranous trachea was preserved. The asterisk indicates the site of membranous trachea resection. An additional 2 cm of membranous trachea was resected (two-headed arrows) and the defect was closed primarily to reduce the length of the defect to 7 cm (right) and 4 cm (left).

TRACHEAL ALLOTRANSPLANT AS CHIMERA

The allotransplant consists of several recipient tissues (1: radial forearm fascia; 2: radial forearm skin; 3: buccal mucosa graft) and donor tissues (4: cartilaginous trachea; 5: respiratory epithelium).

A portion of the cartilaginous trachea was used for **hemilaryngeal reconstruction.**

An additional **strip of forearm skin** was used at the site of membranous trachea resection.

The **cartilaginous trachea** was used at the site with the preserved membranous trachea.

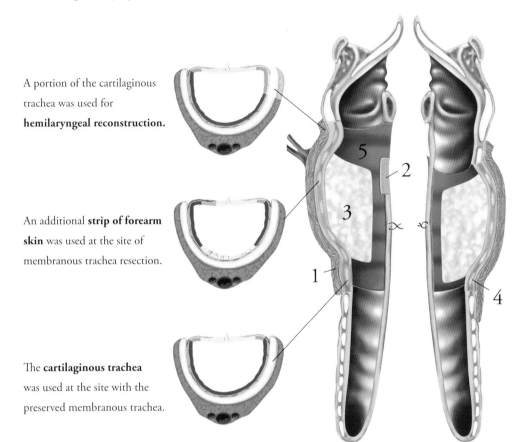

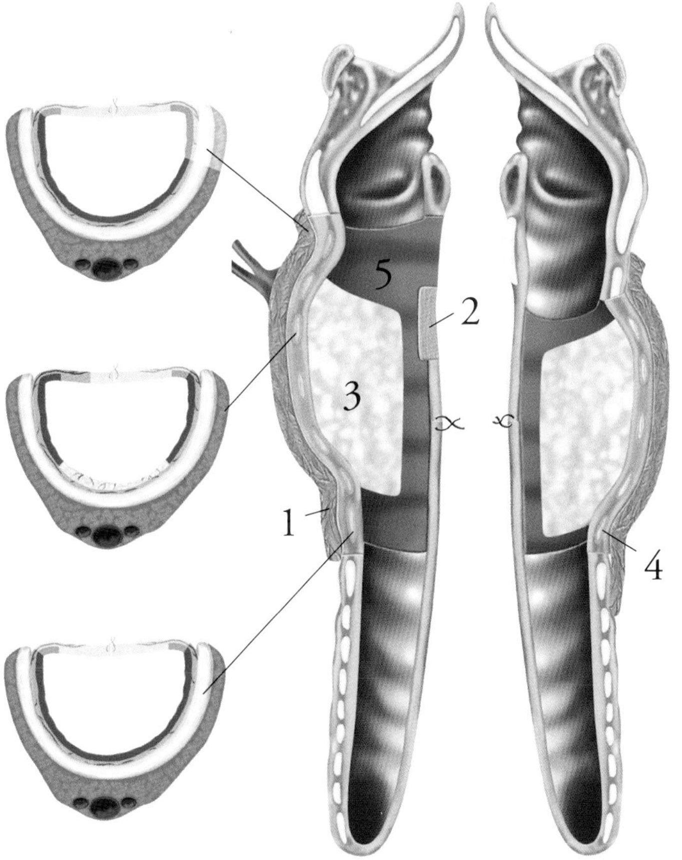
5
2
3
1
4

TRACHEAL ALLOTRANSPLANTATION AFTER TUMOR RESECTION

Tracheal allotransplantation at the time of resection is only possible for low-grade malignancies and not other malignant tumors, because of the risk for tumor progression in the 3-month period of pretransplantation immunosuppression. As a result of the 3-month revascularization and prefabrication period in the forearm, the concept of transplantation appears less suitable for airway correction after the resection of malignant tumors. For tracheal tumors, a temporary reconstruction with a stent surrounded with a vascularized soft tissue flap seems more advisable at this moment (see p. 31). Tracheal allotransplantation may eventually be considered in patients who remain free of tumor.

Tracheal chondrosarcoma - Postoperative CT scan

A CT SCAN TWO MONTHS AFTER ORTHOTOPIC TRANSPLANTATION IS SHOWN. THE TRANSPLANTATION SITE IS VISIBLE ON A SAGITTAL, AXIAL, AND CORONAL CT SCAN.

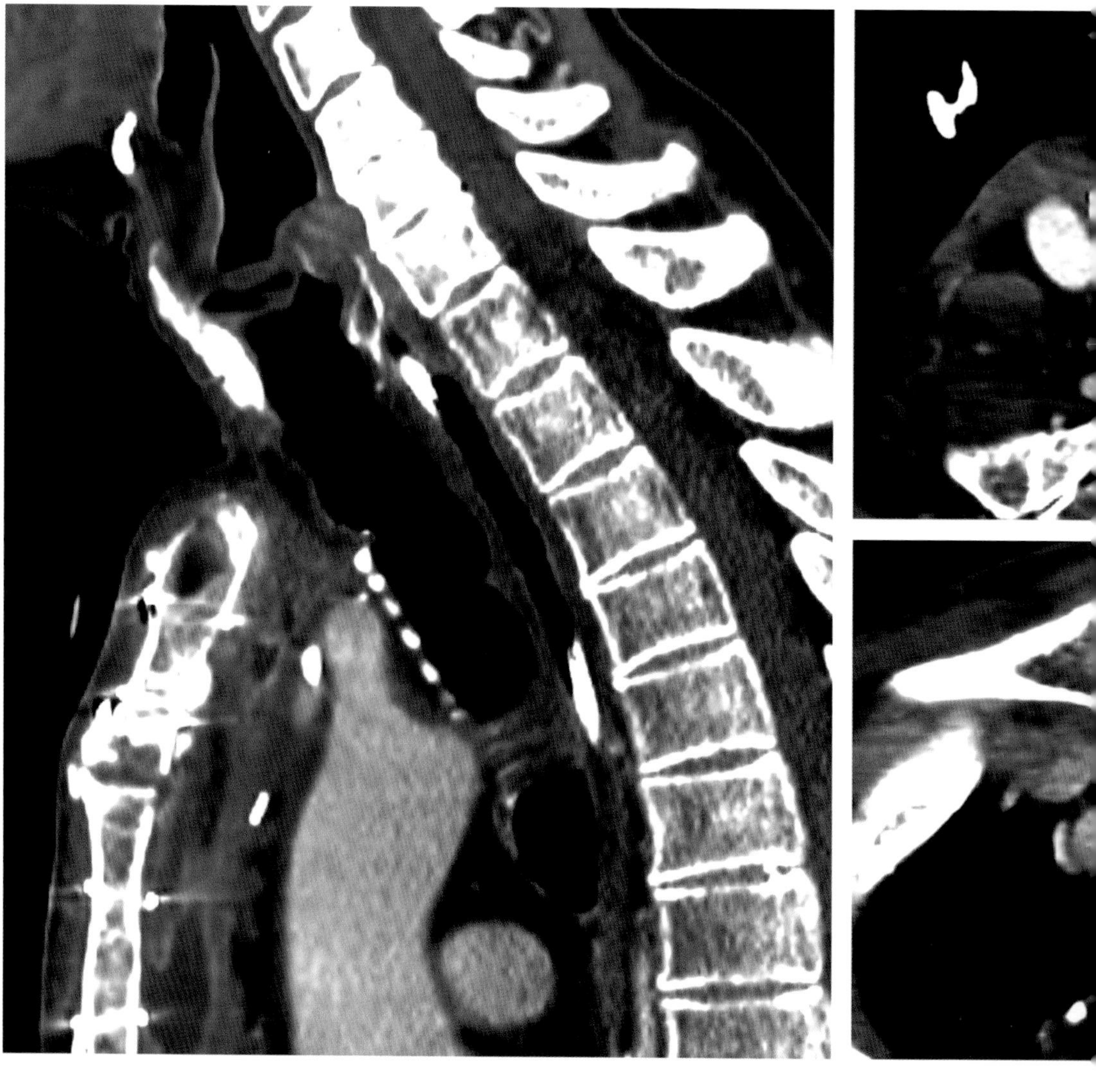

The length of tracheal allotransplant measures 7 cm (right) and 4 cm (left).

"Tracheal allotransplantation at the time of tumor resection is only possible for low-grade malignancies and not other malignant tumors, because of the risk for tumor progression in the 3-month period of pretransplant immunosuppression".

"The anterior incisions of the cartilaginous rings, created at regular intervals to allow for ingrowth of recipient blood vessels, did not disturb the integrity of the reconstructed airway, as all cartilage rings remained intact".

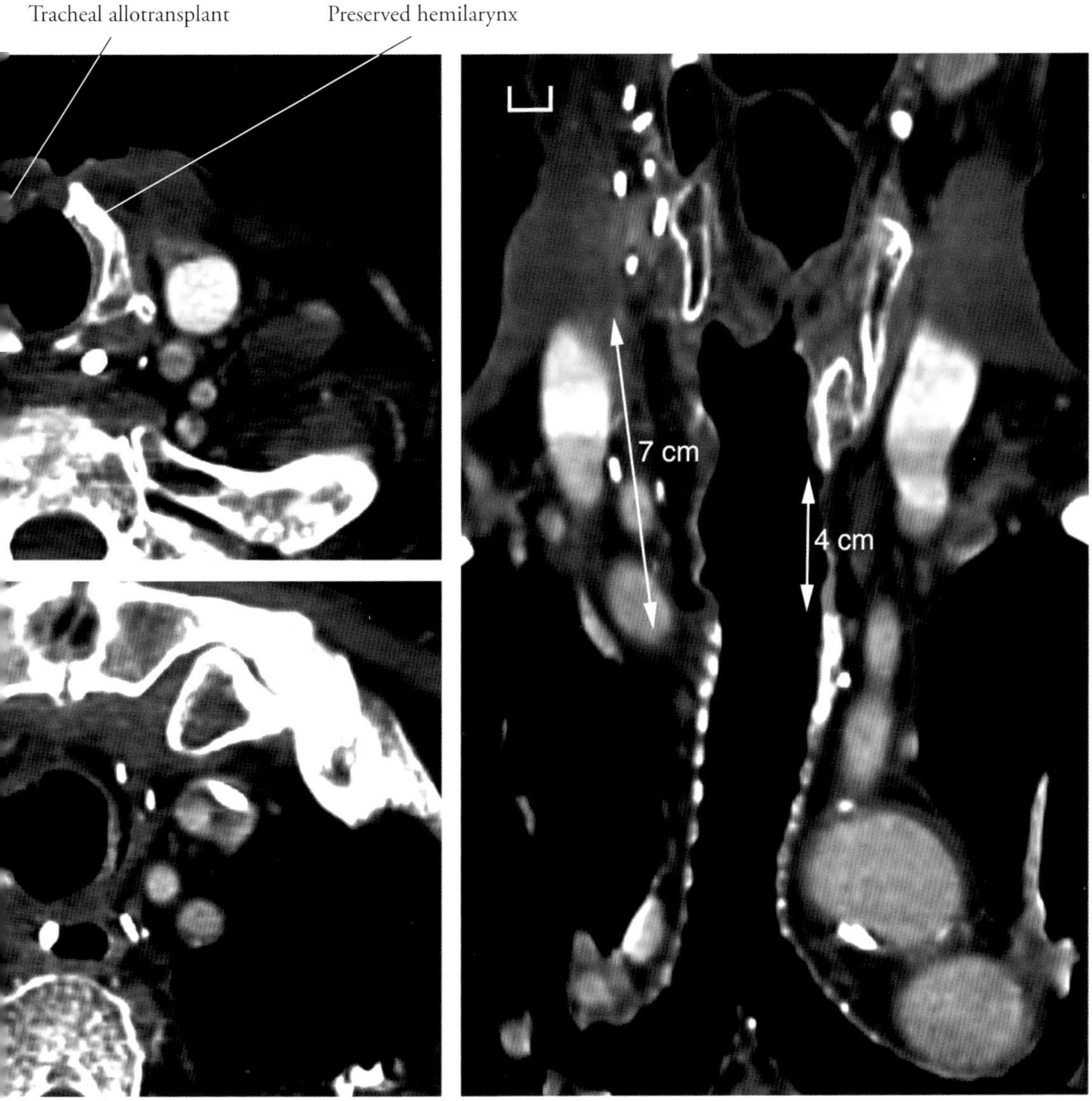
Tracheal allotransplant
Preserved hemilarynx
7 cm
4 cm

Note the absence of cartilage calcification in the allotransplant (scale = 1 cm).

Withdrawal of immunosuppressive medication

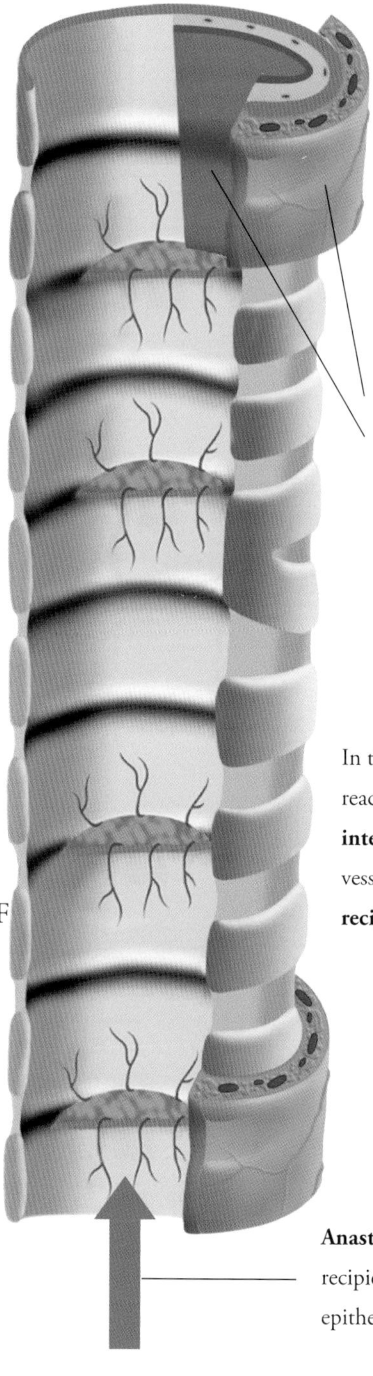

IMMUNOSUPPRESSION

Cartilage is an avascular structure with the chondrocytes protected within a matrix. Cartilage is not rejected by the immune system. To avoid necrosis, the cartilage has to be wrapped in vascularized tissue and the internal site needs a revascularized mucosal lining.

AFTER WITHDRAWAL OF IMMUNOSUPPRESSION

In the **midportion,** recipient blood vessels reach the internal site through the **incised intercartilaginous ligaments.** These blood vessels are necessary for the survival of the **recipient's epithelial lining.**

Anastomotic repopulation by recipient capillaries and recipient epithelium.

IMMUNOSUPRESSIVE MEDICATION WAS GRADUALLY PHASED OUT BETWEEN 12 AND 18 MONTHS AFTER ORTHOTOPIC TRANSPLANTATION. AFTER WITHDRAWAL, A BRONCHOSCOPY WAS PERFORMED EVERY 2 WEEKS. SURVIVAL OF THE MUCOSAL LINING DIFFERRED AT THE ANASTOMOTIC SITES AND AT THE MIDPORTION.

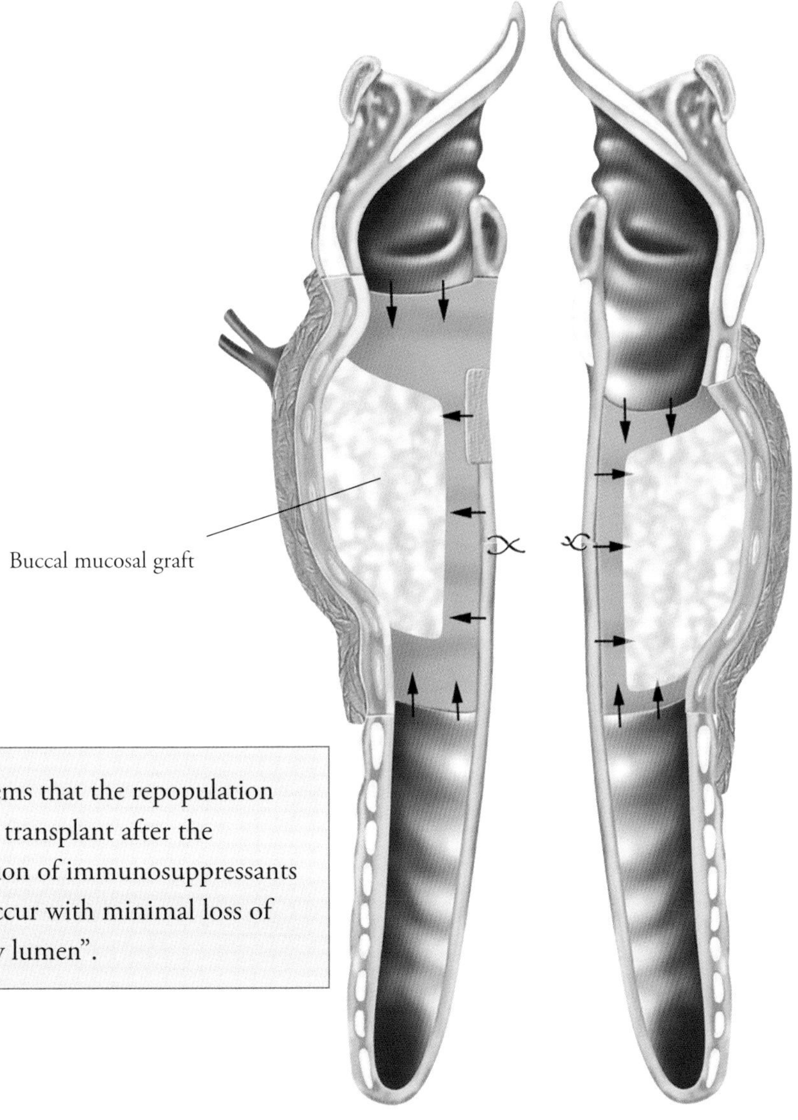
Buccal mucosal graft

"It seems that the repopulation of the transplant after the cessation of immunosuppressants can occur with minimal loss of airway lumen".

Progressive repopulation of recipient endothelium and epithelium at the anastomotic sites (arrows) may have occurred during and after progressive withdrawal of immunosuppressants.

Long-segment stenosis

THE PATIENT INVOLVED WAS A 29-YEAR-OLD MAN. HE SURVIVED THE VOLENDAM FIRE DISASTER (NEW YEAR 2001). HE DEVELOPED A LONG-SEGMENT TRACHEAL STENOSIS DUE TO A COMBINATION OF BURNS AND TREATMENT IN INTENSIVE CARE WITH LONG-TERM INTUBATION. HE FUNCTIONED FOR SEVERAL YEARS WITH A MONTGOMERY T-TUBE. A TRACHEAL TRANSPLANT WAS READY FOR ORTHOTOPIC TRANSPLANTATION THREE MONTHS AFTER FOREARM IMPLANTATION. THE TRACHEAL ALLOTRANSPLANT WAS USED TO AUGMENT A 7-CM LONG STENOTIC LARYNGOTRACHEAL SEGMENT.

BEFORE TRANSPLANTATION

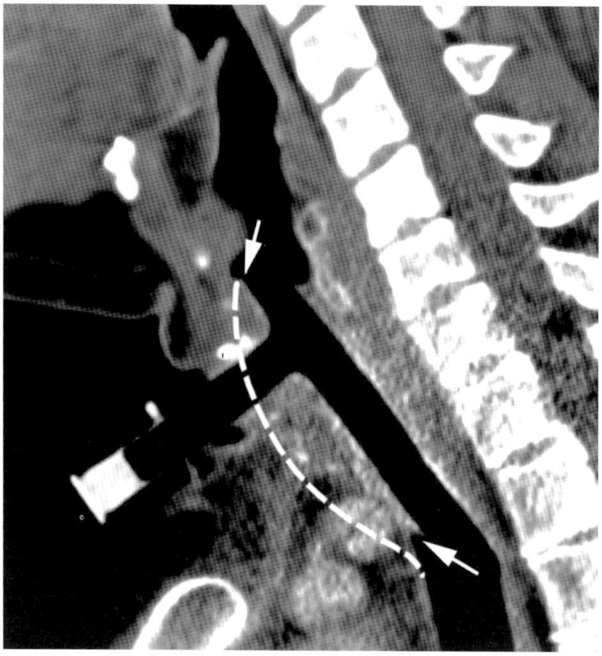

A 7-cm long stenosis of the cricoid and trachea. A Montgomery T-tube (between arrows) was used to bypass the stenosis. The dotted line shows the desired reconstruction area of the airway.

2 MONTHS AFTER TRANSPLANTATION

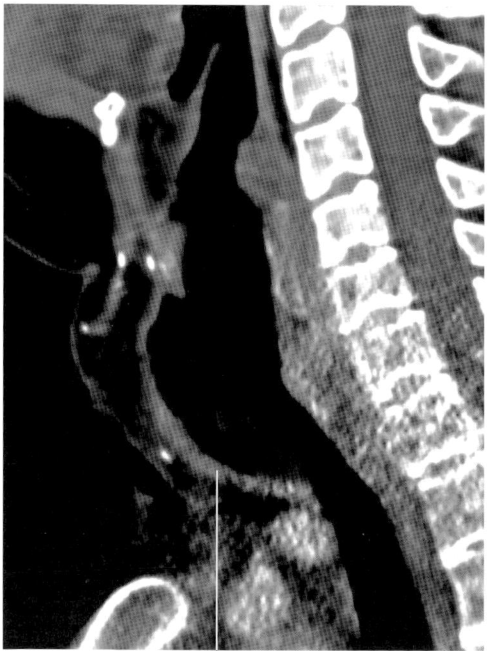

Tracheal allotransplant

Level of the cricoid cartilage

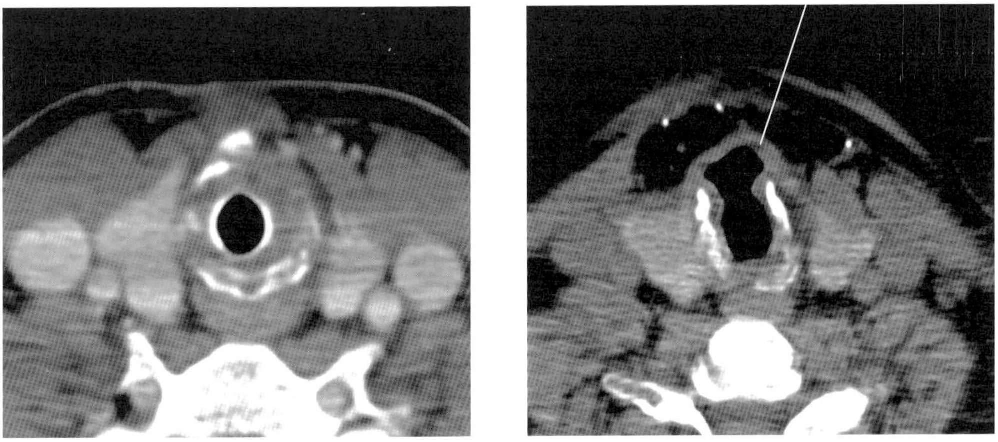
Tracheal allotransplant

Level of the tracheostomy

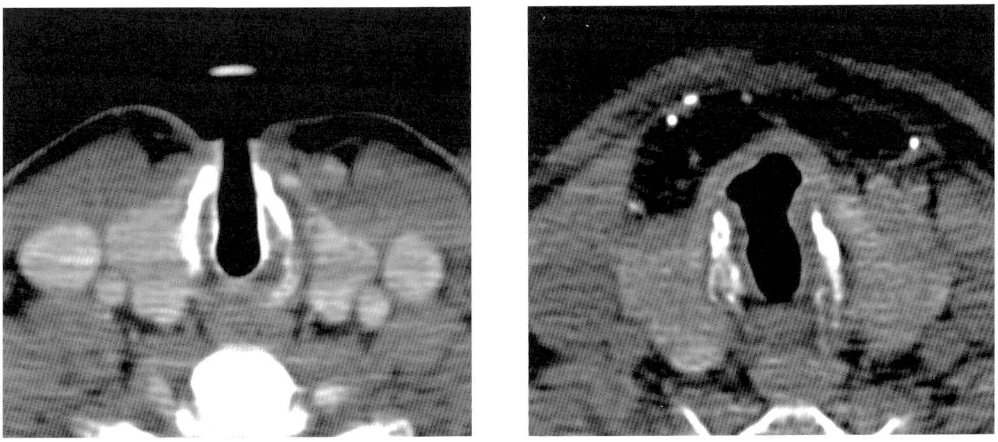

Tracheal level

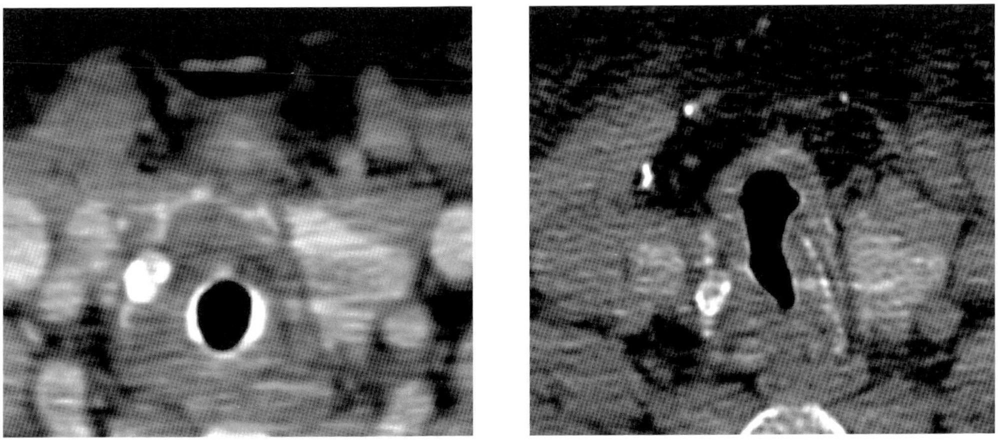

BEFORE TRANSPLANTATION **2 MONTHS AFTER TRANSPLANTATION**

Circumferential reconstruction (1)

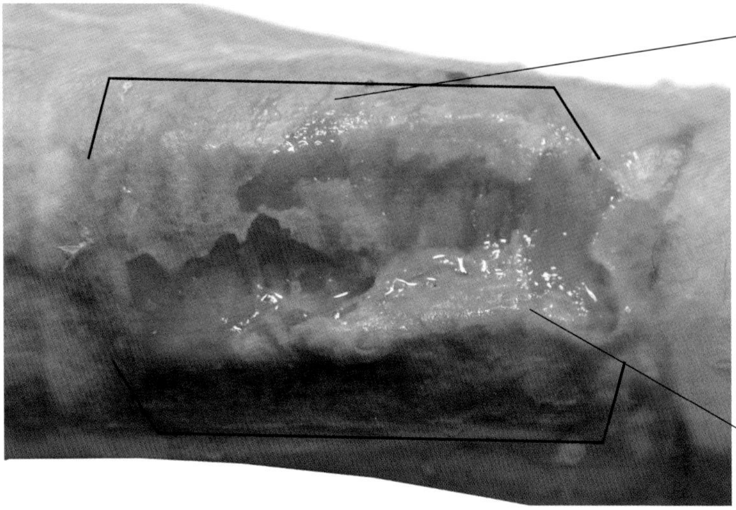

During revascularization, the membranous trachea undergoes necrosis and is replaced by recipient skin.

Vascular connections between the trachea and forearm skin will enable the inclusion of strips of forearm skin for **circumferential airway repairs.**

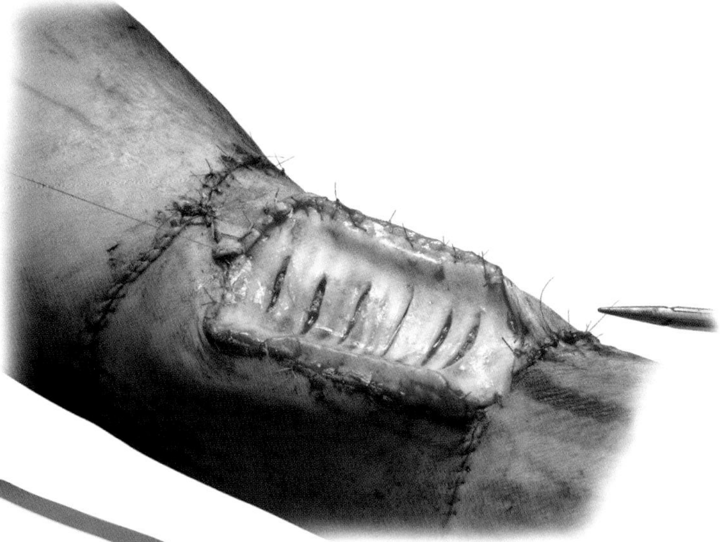

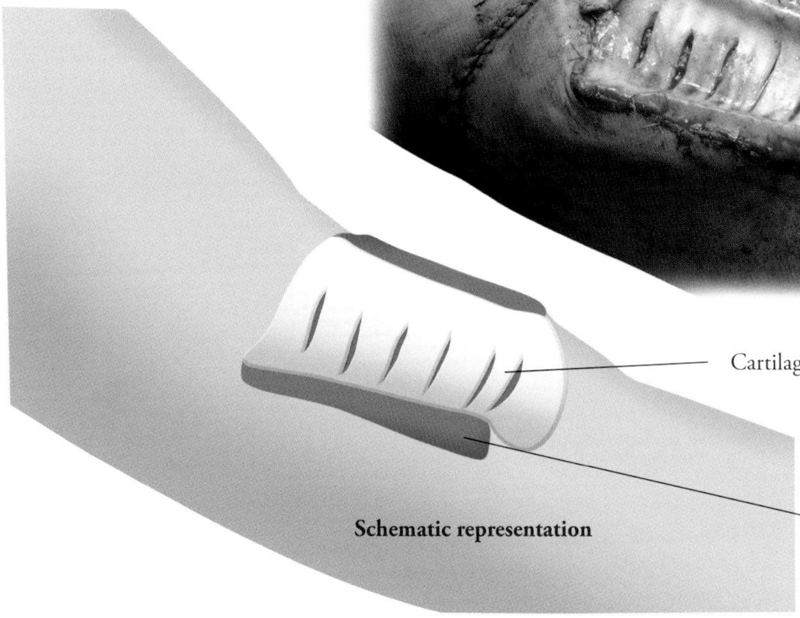
Cartilaginous trachea
Membranous trachea

Schematic representation

A CIRCUMFERENTIAL AIRWAY REPAIR MAY BE NECESSARY AFTER RESECTION OF MALIGNANT TUMORS. THEREFORE, STRIPS OF FOREARM SKIN CAN BE INCLUDED TO FORM A NEW MEMBRANOUS TRACHEA. THE LACK OF SUPPORT WITHIN THE FOREARM SKIN AND THE SWELLING OF THE MUCOSAL LINING AFTER ORTHOTOPIC TRANSPLANTATION WILL RESULT IN A NARROW AIRWAY LUMEN.

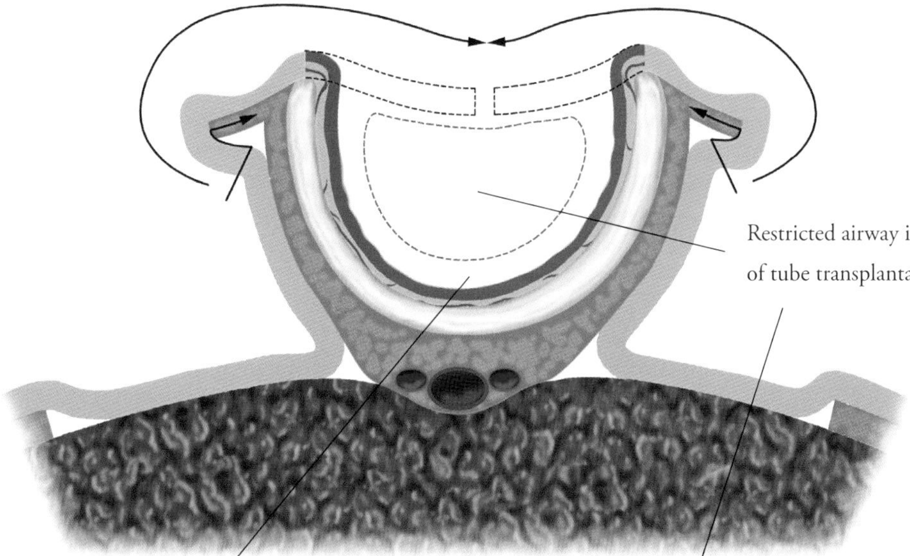

Restricted airway in cases of tube transplantation

Swelling of the mucosal lining during the initial stages of allotransplantation.

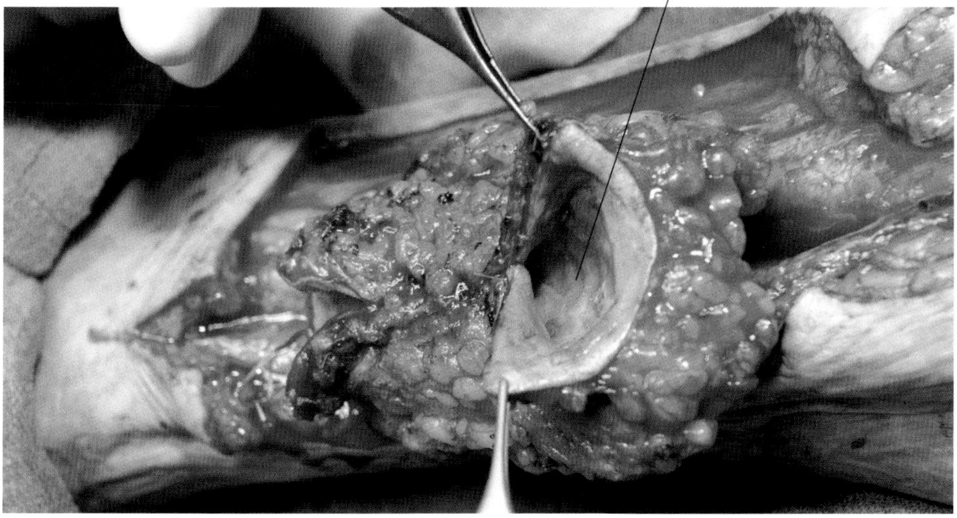

Circumferential reconstruction (2)

FOR CIRCUMFERENTIAL AIRWAY REPAIR, A LARGER AIRWAY LUMEN CAN BE OBTAINED WHEN USING PART OF THE CARTILAGINOUS TRACHEA TO MAKE THE BRIDGE POSTERIORLY. WITH THIS DESIGN, AN 8-CM LONG TRACHEAL TUBE CAN BE CREATED. THEORETICALLY, THE FULL TRACHEAL LENGTH CAN BE REPAIRED WITH THIS AMOUNT OF TISSUE.

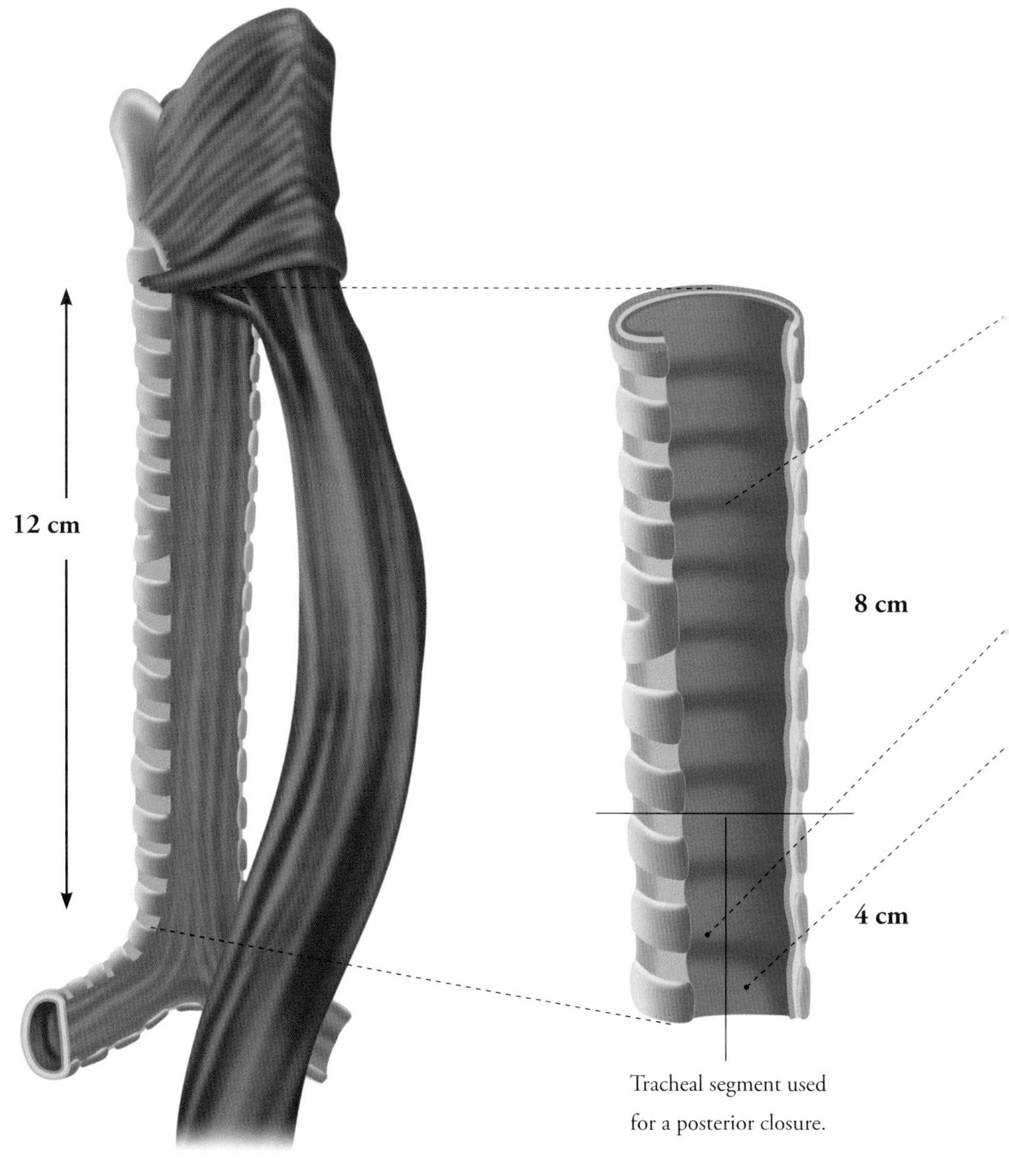
12 cm
8 cm
4 cm
Tracheal segment used for a posterior closure.

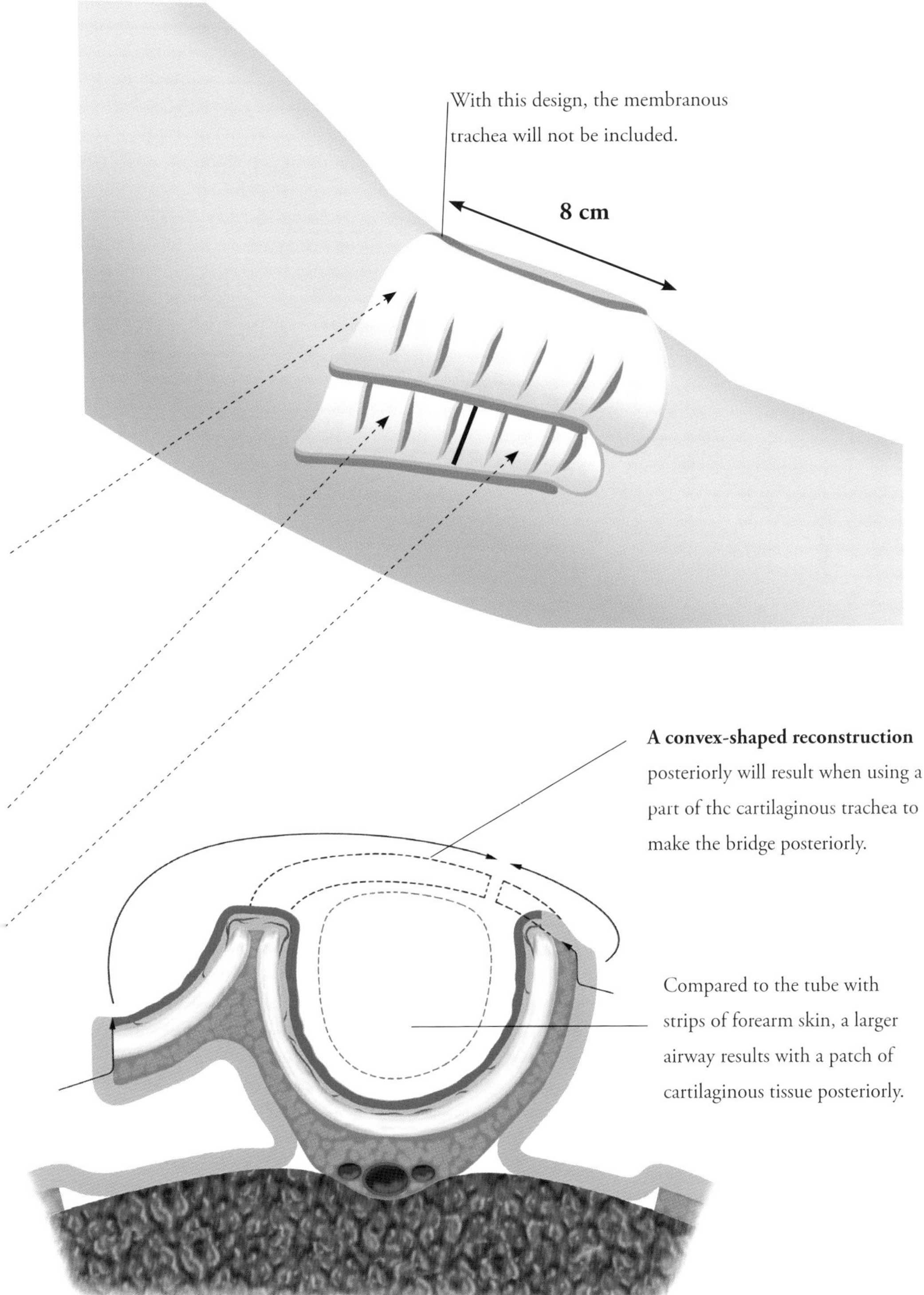
With this design, the membranous trachea will not be included.
8 cm
A convex-shaped reconstruction posteriorly will result when using a part of thc cartilaginous trachea to make the bridge posteriorly.
Compared to the tube with strips of forearm skin, a larger airway results with a patch of cartilaginous tissue posteriorly.

Tracheal allotransplantation - conclusion

THE REVASCULARIZED CARTILAGINOUS TRACHEA IS THE OPTIMAL TISSUE TO REPLACE THE NATIVE CARTILAGINOUS TRACHEA. THIS MAY BE INDICATED FOR THE REPAIR OF LONG-SEGMENT STENOSES.

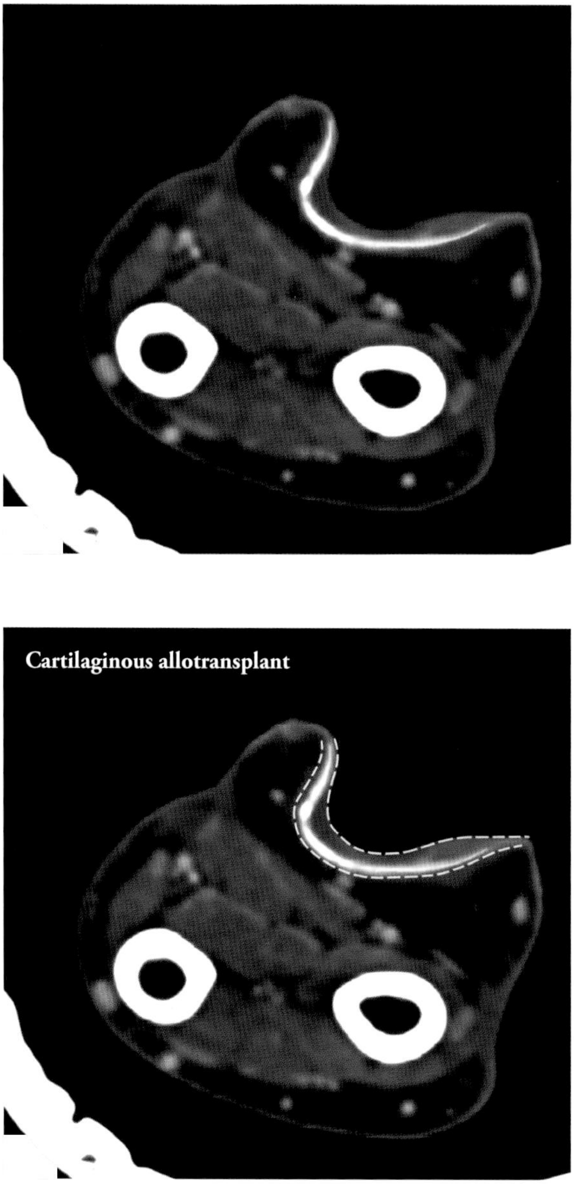
Cartilaginous allotransplant

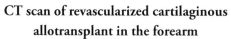

CT scan of revascularized cartilaginous allotransplant in the forearm

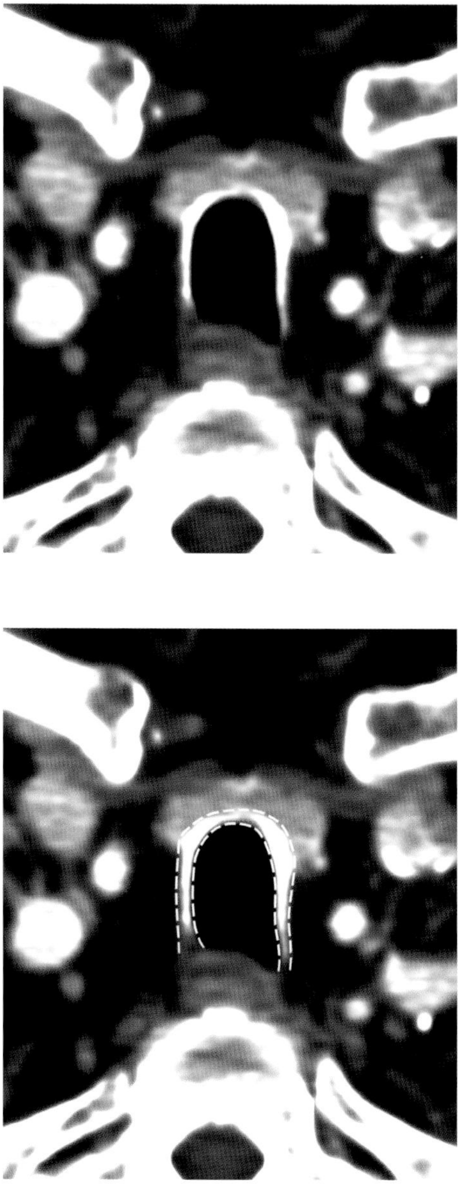

CT scan of the native trachea

TRANSPLANTATION OF A TRACHEAL TUBE MAY BE NECESSARY AFTER A CIRCUMFERENTIAL TRACHEAL RESECTION. A TRACHEAL TUBE CAN BE CREATED BY THE INCLUSION OF STRIPS OF FOREARM SKIN (1). FOR A CIRCUMFERENTIAL REPAIR, A LARGER AIRWAY (2) CAN BE OBTAINED BY USING A PART OF THE CARTILAGINOUS TRACHEA AS A POSTERIOR CLOSURE FOR THE TUBE.

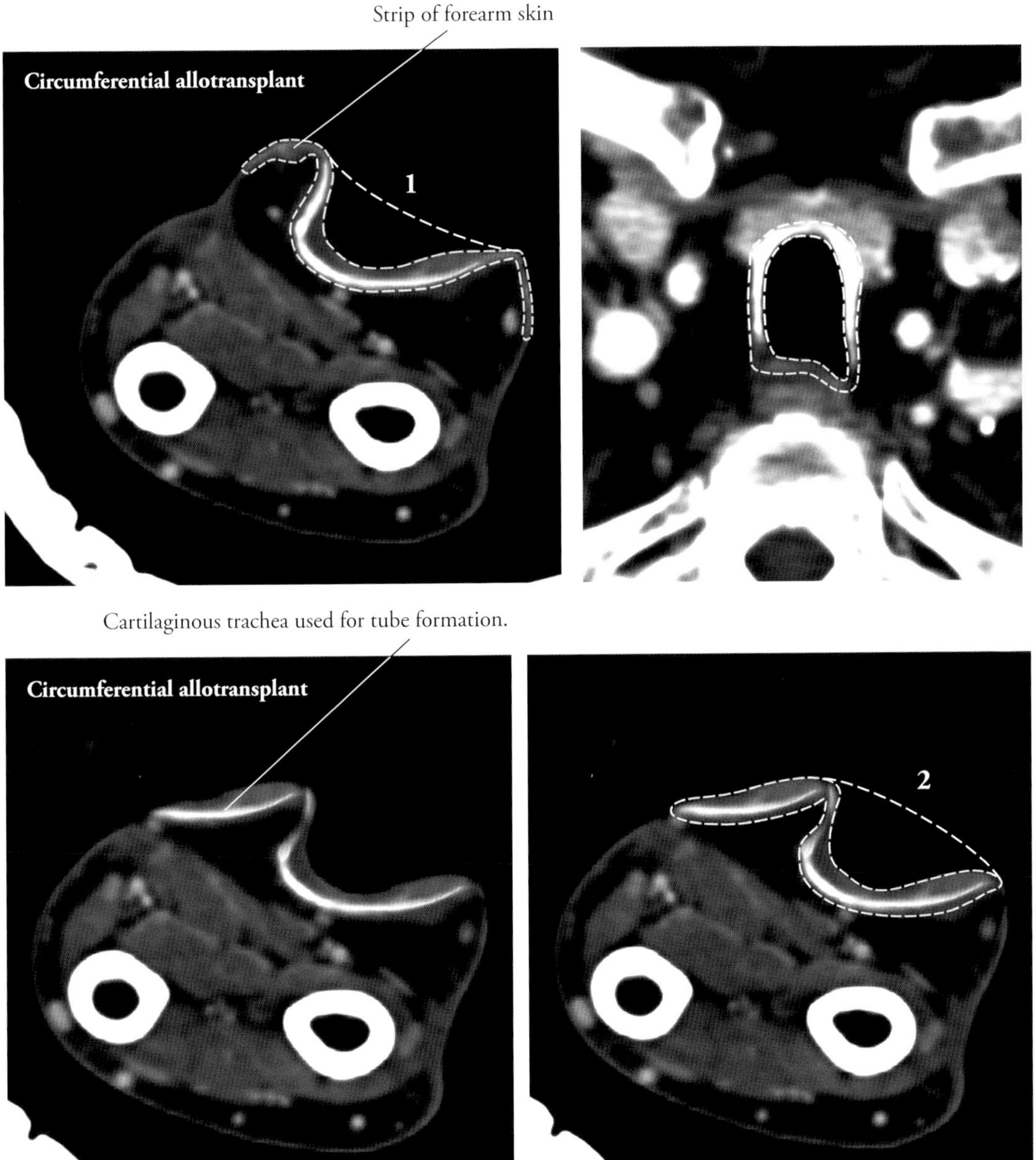
Strip of forearm skin
Circumferential allotransplant
1
Cartilaginous trachea used for tube formation.
Circumferential allotransplant
2

CT scan of revascularized cartilaginous allotransplant in the forearm

CT scan of the native trachea

A sculpture like AGRIEBORZ *not only points to a growing tendency to integrate technology in the human body. It also uses the intriguing possibility to use living tissue as technological material.* AGRIEBORZ *exists in multiple versions: here it is shown as a 3D print (made in collaboration with Materialise, Leuven Belgium).*

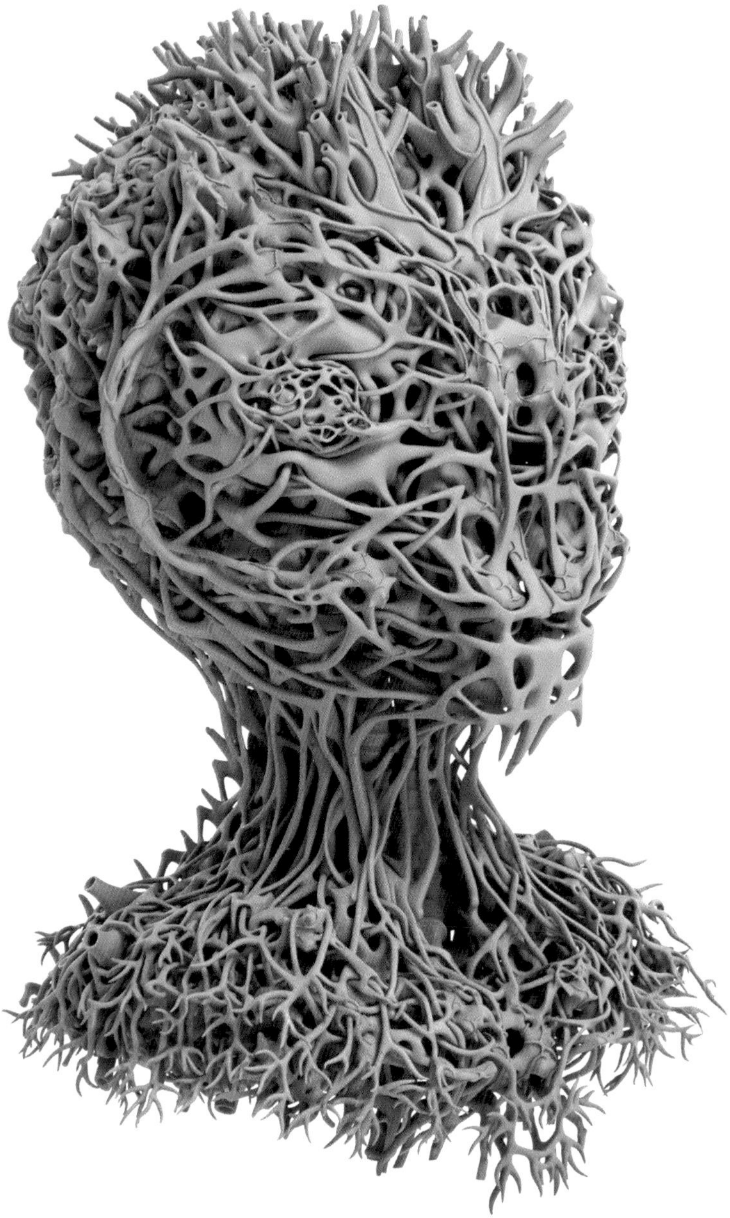

AGRIEBORZ, 2009-2011

3D PRINT – LATERAL VIEW

53 × 34 × 33 CM

Key publications

Delaere P, Ziying L, Pauwels P, et al. Experimental revascularization of airway segments. Laryngoscope 1994;104:736-740.

Delaere P, Ziying L. Tracheal autograft revascularization and transplantation. Arch Otolaryngol Head Neck surg 1994;120:1130-1136.

Delaere P, Liu ZY, Hermans R, et al. Experimental tracheal allograft revascularization and transplantation. J Thorac Cardiovasc Surg 1995;110:728-737.

Delaere P, Ziying L, Sciot R, Welvaart W. The role of immunosuppression in the long-term survival of tracheal allografts. Arch Otolaryngol Head Neck Surg 1996;122:1201-1206.

Delaere P, Vander Poorten V, Guelinckx P, et al. Progress in larynx-sparing surgery for glottic cancer through tracheal transplantation. Plast Reconstr Surg 1999;104:1635-1641.

Delaere P, Hardillo J, Hermans R, et al. Prefabrication of composite tissue for improved tracheal reconstruction. Ann Otol Laryngol 2001;110:849-860.

Delaere P, Hardillo J. Tubes of vascularized cartilage used for replacement of the rabbit cervical trachea. Ann Otol Rhinol Laryngol 2003;112:807-812.

Delaere P, Hierner R, Vranckx J, et al. Tracheal stenosis treated with vascularized mucosa and short-term stenting. Laryngoscope 2005;115:1132-1134.

Delaere P, Goeleven A, Vander Poorten V, et al. Organ preservation surgery for advanced unilateral glottis and subglottic cancer. Laryngoscope 2007;117:1764-1769.

Stamenkovic S, Hierner R, De Leyn P, Delaere P. Long-segment tracheal stenosis treated with vascularized mucosa and short-term stenting. Ann Thorac Surg 2007;83:1213-1215.

Delaere P. Stem cell "hype" in tracheal transplantation? Transplantation 2010;90:927-928.

Delaere P, Vranckx J, Verleden G, et al. Tracheal allotransplantation after withdrawal of immunosuppressive therapy. New Engl J Med 2010;362:138-145.

Delaere P, Vranckx J, Dooms C, et al. Tracheal autotransplantation: guidelines for optimal functional outcome. Laryngoscope 2011;121:1708-1714.

Delaere P, Vranckx J, Meulemans J, et al. Learning curve in tracheal allotransplantation. Am J Transpl 2012;12:2538-2545.

Delaere P. Tracheal transplantation. Curr Opin Pulm Med 2012;18:313-320.

Index

The authors

Pierre Delaere

Born 1959 in Roeselare, Belgium
Professor of ORL - Head & Neck Surgery
University Hospital KU Leuven – Belgium
www.kuleuven.be/cltr

Nick Ervinck

Born 1981 in Roeselare, Belgium
Lives and works in Lichtervelde, Belgium
1999-2001 School of Arts Ghent, Faculty of Fine Arts: 3D
2001-2003 School of Arts Ghent, Faculty of Fine Arts: Mixed Media
www.nickervinck.com

D/2013/45/12 - ISBN 978 94 014 0556 0 - NUR 877

Cover design Paul Verrept
Interior design Jurgen Leemans & Paul Verrept
Artwork Nick Ervinck
Medical artwork Patrick Meeze

Publishing house LannooCampus
Erasme Ruelensvest 179 bus 101
B-3001 Leuven (Belgium)
www.lannoocampus.be